End

When
You
Lose
It

To Adam (Daddy), Ruby Ann & Reva Sam
This is your story as much as ours.
We love you. More than words.

It takes a village.
To all our villagers, we could not have done it without you.
You know who you are.

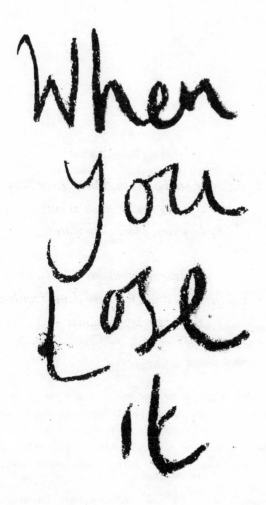

When you Lose it

Roxy + Gay Longworth

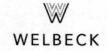

WELBECK

Published in 2022 by Welbeck
An imprint of Welbeck Non-Fiction Limited,
part of Welbeck Publishing Group.

Based in London and Sydney
www.welbeckpublishing.com

A catalogue record for this book is available from the British Library.

ISBN
Hardback – 978 1 80279 218 8

Typeset by seagulls.net
Printed at CPI UK

2 4 6 8 10 9 7 5 3 1

"Some of the names have been changed to protect the guilty."

– Viv Albertine

IN THE BEGINNING

I have been your mother since a watery blue line told me I was. One minute, I am master and commander of my own ship, and then suddenly, I am the ship – and a tiny embryo, deep in the hull, is giving the orders. No two pregnancies are the same, no two births, and no two babies, but make no mistake: mothers are judged as one. I know this because 14 years later, when that thin blue line is hospitalized for suffering a psychotic breakdown, the cross hairs of responsibility perform a rapid sweep of the seascape of your life and quickly lock on their target. The mothership. Me.

One friend, on meeting her child's mental health practitioner for the first time, was confronted with a joke. He said, and I quote,

"You know the old psychiatrist's joke: you're either in here for one reason or a mother."

When you were ill, I had to bang on the door of the mental health services, desperately needing help, tools, skills, advice, compassion, care. Any one of those would have made a difference, yet when I finally rammed my way through, battle weary, exhausted and scared, what I received more often than not was thinly veiled blame. I stood accused. Do they really think that by the time we arrive at their door we haven't already hauled our souls over the hot coals of maternal love? Do they think they are telling us something we don't already fear? I am your mother; of course it's my job to keep you safe. Since you are huddled in the foetal position, rocking at my feet, it is fairly evident I have failed.

I couldn't have loved you more and I am being told that I didn't love you enough, or well enough, or at all. I am your primary caregiver, I am the cause. Already on my knees, heartbroken and wretched with worry, this feels like a cruel blow. And then comes the kicker…

1

"Oh, and by the way, you are the cure as well."

Parenthood is rarely plain sailing. Squalls and storms can descend in the blink of an eye, and even when they have been brewing on the horizon for years, they come as a shock. I know I am not alone, but when the storm hits, I feel entirely and utterly alone. I know you do too. Together, we offer the words of this book as a life raft, a buoy to grab hold of. We would like to help others even though, in the beginning, we could not help ourselves.

This is the story of when I lost you.

1,000-PIECE PUZZLE

To my sisters – I have not been a good sister. I am selfish, uninterested and I have drained our family for years. I am trying to be better. I promise that I will keep trying until I am someone that you can turn to for love and support. You are both such interesting and talented women. You have this strength that I did not have when I was young. You deserved a happy, friendly house to grow up in and I am so desperately sorry that I took that away from you. I am very sorry that I didn't tell you what happened years ago; I hate that you found out through untrue, dramatic rumours. I just wasn't ready to say it out loud. I love you both.

This is going to be difficult to read.

To my dad – I have not been the easiest child to raise. I do not envy you. Thank you for still looking at me like your little girl even when I thought that I was disgusting. Thank you for always believing me.

To the school – you left me alone when I had absolutely nobody on my side. You chose to protect the guilty and put all the responsibility on a 13-year-old girl. You didn't tell the police and you said that was to protect me. You lied to me. I understand that it was too late to really help me, but by protecting the boys, you sent the message to 600 students that what happened to me was acceptable. My maths teacher never should have seen those images.

To the boys – I was 13.

To the reader – when I was just 13, my life fell apart, and I felt like that was it. There was no way I could get out of this. I had just become a teenager and already I did not have the energy to fight. It took me months before I realized that if I was ever going to live the life I wanted, I was going to have to stop punishing myself for what I did, stop hiding out in my house, stop sitting on the sofa wallowing in my all-consuming sadness. It was not easy. It is still not easy. This is the story of how a naive, popularity-obsessed, self-loathing teenager managed to fuck everything up, how life broke her, and how she, with the help of her cold, loving, crazy, indifferent mum managed to put the pieces back together.

This is the story of when I lost it.

To my mum – you are about to find out how little you knew. I hope you are sitting down …

Part 1

TORN

"Get that woman out of there! She needs drugs. Now."

Like a hippo, only my eyes and nostrils can be seen through the matted hair that floats like weeds on the water. The water is cold. I have been in this birthing pool, watched over by a trainee midwife, for – well, to be honest, I don't know, but long enough to contemplate what mercy sinking a few more millimetres beneath the surface would bring. The room glows a handmaid's red. I've no idea what time of night it is, but I do know the man in a suit has just offered me drugs and I am going to follow him.

Sod the lavender oil. Sod the Lamaze breathing. Sod the natural birth. There is nothing natural about this. I rear up. Hurling my distended, white, wrinkled mass out of the birthing pool, I leave a slick of human effluence in my wake, pad out after him, through the double doors, into ...

Oh.

I appear to be in a very busy neonatal ward in a large London hospital. I suppose the architects of the birthing pool room envisaged clean, happy new mothers proudly walking out to waiting family on the other side of the door. At least dry. Certainly robed. Your dad looks surprised to see me, but I don't stop for a chat. I can't lose sight of the man in the suit, so I stride on. He is going to give me drugs. I love him. I feel pretty invincible, but then gravitational force takes on a new meaning and my now upright body restarts the difficult job of cranking itself open to let you out. Instinctively, I drop to all fours and moo like a heifer. I am not sure why your dad is looking so ... nope, I still don't have a word for it.

I look up. I cannot lose the man in the suit, but there are two Emirati men in long white robes getting in my way.

A nurse crouches next to me.

"Are you having a contraction, love?" she asks sweetly, while placing a tea towel over my backside. If you are reading this, sweet nurse, please forgive me for what came out of my mouth.

When the contraction is over, the animal in me gets up, throws off the tea towel and follows in mad pursuit of the man with the drugs. Everyone steps out of my way.

After 36 hours and a failed extraction with a ventouse that pops off your stuck little scalp with such force that the man in the suit, actually now in scrubs, falls off his stool, you are finally delivered by skull-squishing forceps. It doesn't matter because you are out, you are alive and you are beautiful.

"The welts will fade," someone says, "her eyes won't remain bloodshot for long."

What matters is you score 10 out of 10 on your Apgar test. You are perfect. Your dad and I stare at you in wonder, ignoring the man in the scrubs who seems to be taking ages down there, ignoring the fact that it looks like an abattoir in here.

"Just cleaning you up."

He left it to the traumatized trainee midwife to tell me what had happened.

"Third-degree tear," she tells me. I don't know why she is crying; I have a beautiful baby girl.

You lie next to my bed, this tiny, wrapped creature that I know but do not know. Despite being in a deep drug-induced sleep, I am pulled awake. I turn to look at you and these huge dark blue eyes stare directly at me from inside a Perspex box.

"Hello, you."

You blink once, lick your lips and … whoa … you bring forth milk. In that instant, I am reduced to a galley slave and it is your tiny hand now on the tiller, setting the course.

Holy shit, I think, *that is one powerful baby.*

The following day, I feel hot and cold and confused.

"I'm not feeling very well," I try to tell a passing nurse.

"It's just the milk coming in," she says.

"The milk is already—"

But she's gone. In the shower, I discover for myself what a third-degree tear actually means. The wound is infected. I am coming apart at the seam, hole to hole, stitch by nylon stitch. All four layers of them. The stench is indescribable. I hold the stitches in the palm of my hand and show them to the nurse. My temperature spikes to 41°C.

"I could stitch you up again, once the drugs have worked their magic," says the doctor, "but that risks reinfection – better we leave it to heal of its own accord."

"Really? How long will that take?"

"Six weeks," he tells me. "It's a good time to bond with your baby."

The nurses teach me to feed on my side and, awash with antibiotics, we finally go home. Your dad and I take you and a cushion out for supper to celebrate, but it's too much. The only time I sit is in a shallow bath of salt water. I don't really mind, I am so madly in love with your round little face and your round little eyes and your round little nostrils ... you get the gist. First-time mothers. Insufferable.

At the six-week check-up, the wound is still open. I can't really compute how it is okay to leave a new mother with an open vaginal tear and I am beginning to feel crushed by it. Not whole. Torn.

Over the years, I cannot recall how many health practitioners, from conventional to complementary to the downright beardy weirdy, have asked what sort of delivery you had. Forceps, I tell them. "Traumatic" is then duly written next to the word

9

"delivery". I failed. On day one, I failed. I blame myself because back when you were a blue line, the size of a broad bean, I told the obstetric team that I was worried that my insides were oddly shaped. Tampons had always been a problem. I was worried a baby might get stuck too.

"Don't worry," said the male obstetrician, "all women straighten out the same on the day."

I remember feeling a bit belittled when he said it. I wanted to stress my point, but he was the expert and it was rather embarrassing talking about things getting stuck, so I didn't push it. I ignored my own inner wisdom and deferred to a man I had just met and well, you got stuck. I wish I'd stood up for myself. I wish I had trusted my instincts. I missed two vital clues to parenthood. One, children come with their own plan and two, listen to your inner wisdom and trust your instincts even when faced with experts telling you otherwise. Especially when experts are telling you otherwise.

The wound takes six months to heal. The scar tissue knits around the nerve endings, creating a cobweb of pain that requires internal physiotherapy to manually break down. Not as fun as it sounds. The upside is that you and I create an unbreakable bond in our basement bubble. I am stupidly proud of that bond, of the telepathy between us, because it means I can pre-empt your every need. You are rarely fractious and a delightful baby. From six weeks, you are sleeping through the night and we've got sideways feeding nailed. We are two little peas in a tiny pod. Am I smug? Revoltingly so. We are a solid little unit and you are, without exception, my number one priority.

*

"Why do you speak to her as if she understands everything you say?" your dad asks one early autumn afternoon. You have just turned one and are still unsteady on your feet. "She can't possibly understand you."

"Roxy," I say, "go and wipe your sticky hands down daddy's trousers." You toddle towards your besotted father and leave two perfect smear marks down his jeans. That shows him. He can't believe it and, to be honest, even I am a little taken aback. To this day, you know what I am going to say before I say it; you can read my thoughts like ticker tape across my forehead. This is not always a good thing.

*

I believe your troubles start when mine do. We are rushing to catch a Friday commuter train. You are four and have just started primary school. We are pushing your baby sister Ruby in a pram; she is not yet one. I am also pulling a travel cot and carrying a backpack and I have just discovered that I am … I can't even say it. We climb on to the train. It's packed. I haven't got a "baby on board" badge but I clearly have a fair amount of baggage, and no one offers us a seat – why should they? This is entirely self-inflicted. Both my sisters are pushing IVF boundaries trying to conceive and I … Oh God, what am I going to do? I'm not ready. We'll have to move out of our lovely flat. I feel like such an ungrateful shit, but the novelty of pregnancy wears off after the first time. It's boring, I've still got piles, I've got deadlines, I'm clinging on to a career with my fingernails … My husband's life has barely changed, yet mine is unrecognizable. *I* am unrecognizable. The doors start to bleep, they are about to close, I could let go of the little pale hand, the plastic pram, the cot, and jump to the safety of the platform and leave it all behind. I could become a woman I recognize again … They slide shut and lock in place with a hiss. *Oh no, you don't.* I stare at the woman on the other side of the dark glass, the unburdened version of me. *Sorry,* she mouths, and lets me go.

On 10 July 2007, flash flooding causes the Victorian sewage system in the house we have just moved into to catastrophically fail. I am due to give birth in a month. I call my neighbour – please, please, please let our new home be okay.

"It's not good," he says. "Your sofa is floating in 2 foot of raw sewage."

We have no option but to move into a rented house with your newborn sister. Her name is Reva, it means *strength regained,* and it is what I feel the moment she is put into my arms a few hours after she is born courtesy of a stubborn cervical haemorrhage. Overnight, we go from all sleeping on one floor to a tall, narrow house with stairs and landings. You really don't like the house and seem to be reserving judgement on the latest addition to the family. You are the big sister of two babies under the age of two. You look so grown-up next to them. Almost fully formed, except you find it difficult to sleep on your own at the top of this new strange house. I think I know why you're scared. Madeleine McCann's disappearance is on every newsstand we walk by on our way to school. You rarely miss a trick, and you don't miss this.

"It won't happen to you," I tell you.

"But it could."

"It won't."

"It happened to her."

Outsmarted by a five-year-old. In the end, we find a solution. I am up in the night with the baby anyway, so it's best for you to share a room with your dad – then at least not everyone is sleep-deprived. It took six months for the repairs to be done on our house. Sixth months of having the comfort of your protective, generous, kind, doting dad right there with you in the dark.

I realize that two babies in less than two years is a lot for both of us, and you were squeezed out of our pod. One day, I promise you, you will thank me. Unfortunately, only firstborns know what it is like to have an entire cake to themselves. Only they have to watch their cake cut up for a mewling newborn. Only they get to watch, with the hawk-like investigative eye of a toddler, who is getting what slice and how big it is. I tell you this fundamental truth, of which there are very few in this world: each one of you comes with your own cake. You will not know this until you have children of your own. Do you want children of your own? Think carefully: while the love is infinite, time is not. If the firstborn takes up a lot of time, there is less for the second, there is less again for the third, there is very little left for a partner and then there is that job thing, which takes a hefty daily slice. Time gets sliced and diced; it has to be shared. It may be endless, but it has its limits. It flows only in one direction.

*

In 2008, we move into our first proper family home, with a front door of our own. It feels alarmingly grown-up. I have an office at the top of the house and have taken on a new ghostwriting project. Your dad, a theatre producer, is putting on the biggest show of his career and it is exciting. We have three children, so I suppose we are grown-ups now, though I am not sure if I ever truly feel that. I believe I can order the house like my mother ordered ours, but this is not the case. In some ways, I welcome the chaos of three – you just can't get too precious about anything when a baby needs feeding and a toddler needs potty training and the eldest needs to learn her phonetics. I am winging it a great deal of the time. I meet each new challenge, twiddle the dials a bit and hope to evolve. The constantly growing child constantly presents new challenges. That's the thing with firstborns: just when you think you have a handle on the situation, the situation changes. So, it takes quite a long time for me to realize that I have not got a handle on anything when things start to turn sour.

I find myself putting you back into your bed in your room several times a night, night after night. Your little body wracks with fury but I don't really understand why. Bedtime becomes a battleground. By the time you're five, even the build-up to bedtime is a battleground. One evening, I am trying to go out for dinner, and you hang off the front door trying to stop me from leaving. I have to lock you in to stop you from following me. When I do go out, you call incessantly and I try, but fail, to calm you down.

I am watching telly. Footsteps on the stairs.

"I can't sleep," you say.

I wake up in the middle of the night. You are standing next to my bed. Eyes wide, willing me awake.

"I can't sleep."

We try everything. CDs. Audiobooks. Night lights. Poetry. Tickles. Massage. All is calm until the moment comes to actually go to sleep. Then, footsteps on the stairs.

"I can't sleep."

We are locked in a futile battle. I make you go to bed. You can't sleep. You want me to help you sleep, but I cannot. I tell you to stay in bed, because you sure as hell won't fall asleep crouched on the stairs hoping I won't notice you. Nothing works.

Eventually, I take you to the doctor. He says it is developmental, separation anxiety possibly brought on by a new school, new house, new siblings, new childminder. He reassures me it is perfectly normal in a four-year-old. You're nearly six.

SLEEP TIGHT

You are going out for dinner. You go out for dinner as much as possible – you don't want to be around me in the evening.

Sometimes I try to stop you. Tonight, I want everything to be okay. It is Ruby's birthday tomorrow. I am willing myself to stay in control, to not let my brain win. Tonight will not be like last night. As soon as I sit down for dinner, the fear starts to creep in. It isn't overwhelming; small lapses of concentration, a slight shake in my left leg, my teeth clawing at my bottom lip until it bleeds. I do everything that I am supposed to do. I take 10 of the crystal drops that the man with the long white beard gave me. I try to breathe slowly and deeply – everybody says that will help; it hurts my chest and makes me feel so completely out of control of my own body.

I go to my room and start my routine, my ritual. I check the cupboards, the drawers, under the bed, make sure the window is locked – standard stuff. I measure the door; it has to be open about 3 inches wide so that I can see one of the lights on the corridor and 10 of the stripes on the corridor carpet, but not so wide that I can see any of the stairs.

I read. I get through a book about every two days. I read until my eyes go blurry, until I am so exhausted that surely I will fall asleep when my head touches the pillow. I turn the light off and sprint across the room to bed. As soon as the lights turn off, my brain starts to whizz again. I am suddenly wide awake, on edge, and the aching fear that I am going to die tonight takes over.

I turn on an audiobook and I stare at the three inches of light coming through the door. I try to force my brain to focus on the words of *The Railway Children*, but it is more like I am being told what to think rather than me doing the thinking. I have to write it down. I have to write it all down, otherwise I will forget, and I cannot forget. Pages of scribbled notes cover my bedside table, and I often wake up in the morning with no recollection of writing these pages and pages of thoughts.

I hate myself for not being asleep, and I start to get more and more nervous that I am getting to the end of my audiobook. With every minute, I get a little more terrified that the CD is coming to an end, so I rewind every five minutes.

I think that I am going to die. I don't know how, but it is going to happen.

I bite my nails, and then add them to my collection of nail ends.

I scribble more notes and rewind my tape and wait for the sound of the front door.

I look out of the window for anything suspicious. I am not sure what would count as suspicious, but I think that I will know when I see it.

I hear the front door, but there is a voice in my head telling me that it isn't you, that somebody else has come into the house. I sneak downstairs, just to check.

"Mummy, I can't sleep."

You look as exhausted as me. I go up to bed, and then back down to your room, then back to bed, then back down to your room, the back to bed, then ... your bedroom is locked. You have locked me out. I think that I am about to die and you have locked me out. You are not going to protect me or save me – you don't want me anywhere near you. I am in danger and you are behind that door ignoring my screams.

I bang on your door because somebody is coming to get me.

I need backup, so I wake up Ruby.

"We are in danger, we need help and Mummy has locked us out."

I take a broomstick and I start to bang on the door. We are in danger. We need help.

Then your face is in the doorway. You are now scaring me more than my previous fears. It's your eyes that destroy me; they are so full of anger and hatred. When we go to your friends' houses, I see the way you look longingly at their children, wondering why you didn't get that.

There is more screaming and shouting. You are angry at me – you think that I am attention-seeking and should be punished. Why can't you see that this is awful for me too? Don't you think that I wish I could sleep? I am exhausted and I am never safe. You think that I don't want all this to stop?

Eventually, I am curled up on the sofa at the end of your bed. Finally, I can sleep.

In the morning, I am so sorry. I cannot believe it happened again. I promise that it will be the last time. I walk into my bedroom and it seems so unthreatening. Of course I am safe here – it is pretty ridiculous that anybody could be hiding in my cupboard. Tonight will be different. Tonight, I will be easy.

I write you a sorry card for you to add to the collection stacked up next to the fridge. It is the fourth one this week. It is too late, though. I have ruined Ruby's birthday. It isn't the last time.

SUGAR AND SPICE

School is the other battleground. Morning after morning, you dig in your heels and I find myself physically dragging you along the grey, chewing-gum-pockmarked pavement, with you in full-blown tantrum mode while I'm pushing your two sisters in a double buggy. It's not a good look and I am ashamed to say I feel embarrassed. Why can't you happily skip along next to me like everyone else on the busy school thoroughfare? Why the scene? By 8:30 in the morning, I feel broken.

One day, you come back from school.

"Mummy, what's a freak?"

Hmm. I go in to talk to your teacher. She says she will keep an eye on you and reports back that you appear to be very happy at school. There are no concerns. Indeed, when I arrive back at the school gates, you are frequently the last to the door, taking one look at me and then running back into the building, often with the girl who you've told me is being mean to you.

"No one plays with me at break."

"Why don't you ask the girls if you can join them?"

"I do. They say I have to ask the person who started the game, so I ask the next girl and she says I have to ask the girl who started the game, so I ask the next girl and she says …"

I get it.

"What about four-square?" I ask. You just look at me with disdain. Let me explain the subtle changes of the rules of four-square depending on who is playing it. In this case, you. You queue for ages to get a turn to replace the girl who has dropped the ball. Finally, you are in the square and the ball gets thrown hard at your chest; you don't catch the ball and go back to the end of the queue. Not all girls are sugar and spice. I go back to the teacher.

"Well, you know what girls are like," she says.

I'm sorry, what?

Perhaps if girls were allowed to bash it out in the yard like the boys do and work out supremacy that way, they wouldn't need to be so conniving. But girls are supposed to be "good".

Their tactics require a magician's sleight of hand, which means you keep getting sawn in half.

Eventually, we go and talk to the head.

"Well, you have been away working a lot," says the female head of a girl's school.

To which my loyal husband replies, and for this and a million other things, I will be forever grateful: "She has, but I've been here."

The woman observes him with quiet pity. It was not the help I was hoping for.

THREE-SQUARE

I cannot go to school. I haven't slept. I am so tired. You are angry at me, but I need you.

The walk to school is not long enough. I slow down as we get to the streets near the entrance. I pray that the traffic lights are red so that we can wait for longer at each crossing.

The teachers at the school gate smile sweetly and welcome me in.

Please do not leave me here. Don't let their smiles trick you.

I like the lessons where all the desks face the front. I can lose myself in the lesson and forget about the people around me. These people who are supposed to be my friends, or at least my peers, seem so alien to me. It feels like they are just living in a completely different world. I hate the lessons where we sit around tables facing each other.

When the bell for morning break rings, I race to the library. I find a corner and open my book, my shield. There are few books left in this library which I haven't read. The librarian gives me some shelves to organize, an invaluable distraction.

As soon as the lunchtime bell rings, I am back at the library door.

"I'm sorry, Roxy. I have a meeting today, so the library is closed. It is a beautiful day, go and play outside."

No. No. NO. My fingers are at my mouth and I am ripping at the skin.

With my heart rate racing, I join the queue for four-square. Four people stand in a square and bounce the ball to each other. The person who loses control of the ball is kicked out and replaced by the person at the front of the queue. The conversation in the queue is like a different language to me and I cannot translate. I eventually get to the front of the queue.

"Sorry, we are actually now playing three-square, so there is no room for you."

Do not cry, Roxy. Do not cry. Crying will make it so much worse. I practically run to the bathroom, leaving the laughter behind me. I wait in the bathroom, longing for the bell to ring again.

It is finally the end of the day, and I am packing up my bag. Two girls come up to me. *Please don't talk to me.*

"If you tense your stomach, then you won't feel it when we punch you."

"Sorry, my mum is waiting for me, I really need to go."

"Come on, don't be a freak. Tense your stomach when we get to three. One ... Two ..."

They punch me.

"I wasn't ready," I splutter, but they have already run off laughing.

You are waiting for me at the gate. I can't come home. Home means bedtime, and sleep, and fear, and you being angry at me, and me being angry at myself. I hide behind the pillars in the school entrance. I don't want to go home.

*

You are going out tonight, so our babysitter is here. She doesn't understand this scary world inside my head either. She is a large, elderly, very Catholic Filipino woman called Fatima. My youngest sister is her baby, but she thinks that I am too far gone to be helped. Nevertheless, she is trying to cleanse me of the devil inside. I am only eight. I don't understand why the devil wants to be inside me. There is a shelf in my room holding the figurines Fatima has brought back from her various pilgrimages.

She comes to turn my light off with a bottle of holy water in her hand. She dips her finger into the bottle and draws a cross on my forehead. She says that I am possessed by Satan, but that there is a good girl inside.

I know, Fatima; I am also trying to find the good girl inside.

Right now, every ounce of strength I have is going in to stopping my brain from running away with whatever terrifying thought comes into my mind. I scribble some more notes on the paper next to my bed. Important things that I desperately need to tell you.

Fatima sits by my bed and prays with me. Or prays for me – I don't quite know.

REGRESSION

I am in my office late, alone, lying on the floor thinking about you while a woman halfway across the world is tapping into our higher selves.

"I have regressed your past lives," says the woman in California. Of course she is from California. While I am naturally a sceptic, I am also desperate. She comes highly recommended by a friend who used healers when her son was diagnosed with a rare form of cancer. He is now in remission, so I am ready to take the leap. I want to believe. So I believe. Isn't that the definition of faith?

Why am I lying on the floor following a guided meditation by a spirit healer on an international call? Well, after a miserable summer full of escalating friction between us, I asked my family what I should do. Their answer was succinct and unanimous: "Get professional help."

So I did. A GP referred us to the Tavistock Institute for family therapy, but your dad is unsure. He was referred to a therapist when he was a teenager, and all they did in their sessions was smoke. A child psychiatrist told me you had transitional issues – school to home, day to night – and a very active imagination, both of which I agree with. He referred us to a child psychologist, who told us you are a very bright little girl who doesn't like school.

Yes, yes, but when are we going to get advice? What can help?

A clinical psychologist told me to regain control of the household. A tyrant – you – is in charge, and I am letting the tantrums rule. The key here is your fear of sleep. Every time I give in to the fear – and let you sleep with me or your dad – I am inadvertently telling you there is something to be afraid of, therefore allowing the obsession, a fear of sleep, to be appeased by the compulsion, staying awake. What I must do is hold the line and tell you there is nothing to be afraid of, and in the morning show you the proof. You are alive. This is the way neural pathways in your brain start to realign, by challenging the obsessive thinking and resisting the compulsion.

But I have done this, I beg the psychologist to understand, a million times, and it just leads to tantrums. Nothing seems to tire you out. I, however, am permanently knackered. I don't know what I am supposed to do – I can't physically restrain you. The clinical psychologist suggests I put a lock on your door. Instead, I put a lock on mine. You try and break through the door with something; I don't know what you are using, as I don't give in and I don't open the door. Eventually, it stops and I assume you are curled up outside the door, spent. Perhaps it is the only way you can sleep. It is not a night I wish to repeat, so I continue my search to understand why you can't stay in your bed like all the other kids I know. And that search has led me to a woman in California.

By now you are eight and, after four years of this, I am desperate. The lady in California speaks again:

"You and Roxy are in a cave in the Afghan mountains …"

Okaaay …

"You're dead. She is alone in the cave, it is pitch-black and you have left her all alone—"

"Hang on, I'm dead? Surely you can't—"

She cuts me off.

"Doesn't matter. She is a child, and you are supposed to be looking after her, but you've left her in a cave, alone. She's terrified, and you're no comfort."

I feel terrible. I am lying on my bed communing with a woman in California for a fairly hefty price who has just told me I am as comforting as a corpse. The thing is, something is ringing true, but I can't quite put my finger on it. I really do feel terrible sadness for this child in the cave.

Wake up, Mummy, wake up.

But I can't wake up. I'm dead to the world.

Why am I dead to the world? Because I am so fucking exhausted.

The Californian woman's voice softens.

"Look, Gay, it doesn't matter if you don't believe me, just know that when your daughter is alone in the dark, that is how frightened she feels."

I paid with gratitude and something very precious: at last, a glimmer of understanding. Your dad finds me crying in the bath and I tell him everything, like I always do. I'm not crying from sadness, weirdly. I'm crying because I finally know what you are feeling and as mad as it sounds, it is the first time I feel on solid ground. I have a vivid imagination. I can still see that child in the cave next to her dead mother, draped in darkness and terror. Your fear is real to you. I don't know why you're afraid. But I know you're afraid.

I have your room "cleared" just in case. You are given blue bottles of tinctures which I drop on your tongue. I try homeopathy. Neither work. You are immune even to the placebo effect. You are still afraid, and still you don't sleep.

*

It is a beautiful blue-sky day and we are walking around a small school in the country about 45 minutes from where my mum grew up. Boys and girls run around an open field; the sound of laughter carries across the soft summer breeze. You are in deep conversation with the head teacher, who is showing us around acres and acres of outside space.

"So when are you thinking of coming here?" he asks you.

"As soon as possible," you reply.

Ouch.

"No, no," we laugh, "This would be for when you leave primary school." You're only nine.

"She could come now," says the head. "We offer boarding to a small number of children who live far away."

24

Your dad and I look at each other. But not 140 miles away, surely?
But you – you are adamant.

"I would like to come now." You look at me. "I don't want to stay at my school."

School has been an uphill battle, we've made it through, but with a lot of scaffolding. There isn't a book in the library that you haven't read. You've been on some kind of supervision for a while now and I've taken a sabbatical to join the super-involved PTA just so I could get on the inside and see for myself what was going on in the corridors after you told me you were punched in the stomach. Still, I don't want you to get your hopes up, and despite all our problems, I don't want you to be so far away. That feels like a failure. Like I can't look after my child.

"You have to get in first," I warn.

"She'll get in," says the head.

On the way home, I start to imagine a new way of life for you and us: no more bedtime squalls, some breathing space for everyone, more time for your sisters, your dad and I being able to share a bed, uninterrupted sleep, routine for you, cozy bunk beds, a dorm – you'd never have to sleep alone – and new friends made outside the shark-infested waters of a high-pressure feeder school. Maybe it isn't such a mad idea to be in a softer school, known for its generous pastoral care.

Your London school was very outcome-focused. I once asked a mother why the girls were doing times tables in reception. You were four years old at the time and it seemed a bit harsh to me. She explained that by teaching the curriculum two years ahead of schedule, they got the girls into the best secondary schools, which then got them into Oxford or Cambridge where – and I quote (I shit you not), "they'll meet the right sort of man". Perhaps I should have taken you out then and there. Later on,

I was worried that you might take the problems settling in to your peer group with you. I believed it would serve you better in the long run if you worked out the issues first, then left on your own terms if you wanted to. You had done this and I was proud of you for that. You had a small group of sweet friends. Now the only thing looming on the horizon was the dreaded secondary school entrance exams.

By switching systems, we could bypass all that and you'd be able to stay at the new school until you were 13. In the end, I think this is what swings it for me. Entering secondary school having just turned 11 would feel like feeding you to the wolves all over again. By the time we get home, it's decided. You will weekly board and we will rent a converted barn near my parents and spend the weekends in the countryside. I am really excited for the first time in years.

When you arrive, you sleep with three hockey sticks and have to face the door so you can keep watch for predators. Eventually, three hockey sticks become two, then one, then none. You still need to be able to see the door, though you never tell me why.

"I wish I was brave like you," you say.

"I'm not brave, my angel, I'm just not scared. It's not the same thing."

You have just turned 10, you're 140 miles away from us, you know no one, you've left the city in which you were born, and yet you think you aren't brave? Sweetheart, you are one of the bravest people I know.

People warn me that sending a child to boarding school is like a bereavement. I will be absolutely honest and tell you this is not the case for us. We still have long phone calls in the evenings with you, and settling in takes a while. Friendship issues linger, but things are easier at home and your sisters are allowed to be happy-go-lucky children without the spectre of nightly rows and combative journeys to school. You come out every weekend, and we get spoilt with your dad's best cooking, light fires, watch *Strictly*, take muddy walks to the pub, go for tea with my parents. We have fun in short, manageable bursts and it's only one night, so you can sleep with whomever you like. At school, you discover you're smart and good at sports. It works for you, so it works for us. I think it was one of the few good decisions I made.

HOCKEY STICKS

I am nearly 10 and have decided that I cannot live like this any more. The fear, the exhaustion, the feeling that I am ruining my family, the fact that you hate me. I do not want to be here any more, I cannot be here. So I ask you if I can go to boarding school, and you let me. Of course you let me; you don't want me here any more either.

I sleep in a dormitory with six other girls. I love that I never have to sleep on my own. I love the fire and smoke alarms in every room. I love the fire escape routes stuck up in every room, and the CCTV cameras. I love that there is a plan.

Night after night, I lie in bed and will myself to fall asleep before the older kids come to bed. I can't still be awake when everyone has gone to bed. My old iPod plays the only album that it has downloaded: *All I Intended to Be* by Emmylou Harris. Halfway through the album, my heart starts to speed up. Why am I still awake? The album is coming to an end. My head is spinning and I beg the songs to go slower. I repeat the penultimate song six times.

Go to sleep, Roxy.

I ponder over the probability that I am the only person awake in the whole building. Eight dormitories, at least four beds in each room, plus the teachers who live here. Surely, surely, I am not the only person awake at this horrible hour. My brain has taken over and I am being dragged into very dark places. How are all these girls sleeping peacefully when something so bad could happen the second I fall asleep? Asleep, I have no protection and nor does anyone else. You are so far away. I know that there is a box downstairs full of old hockey sticks. I sneak downstairs and then I am back in bed with a hockey stick tucked up safely next to me. Just in case. The next night, there are two hockey sticks in my bed. This happens every night.

On Saturday afternoons, you pick me up and take me to a barn you've rented so that we can all spend the weekends together. I sleep with you, and because I am only home one night a week, you let me. This is a huge relief, because the barn is scary. Huge glass windows that just lead to blackness. Nothing and nobody around for miles. Cheap wooden doors that don't lock. So much glass. We had to flick mouse poo off the pillows before bed, and in the morning, I would wake up with brick dust on my face from the walls. The nights are less bad now because I don't see you very much, so we try to make it special. You are nicer to me. During the holidays, it sometimes slips back to how it used to be, with the fear and the anger and the lack of understanding. If you don't want me to sleep with you, things go badly.

I am sleeping on my own tonight. I am going to sleep on my own the whole night through and you will be proud of me in the morning. I count the bricks on the wall opposite the bed. Then I count only the horizontal bricks. Eventually I do fall asleep which, in itself, is a huge achievement. But in my sleep, there are gorillas who are breaking into the house. One rips my bedroom door off so that it is hanging off one hinge. The gorilla scratches and hits the door. It screams at me and runs out. I run across the dark, unprotected landing to your bedroom. I shake you to wake you up. You and dad are lying dead in bed next to each other.

I wake up. The door is not ripped off, but there are darks marks on it that I swear were not there before. I make the terrifying trip across the landing and shake you as hard as I can to check that you are okay. You are alive but not happy to see me and not relieved that I have survived the gorilla attack.

"Go back to bed. We can talk about your bad dream in the morning."

It took all the strength I had to cross the landing alone to get to you. There is absolutely no way that I can go back to my room. I know you are sleepy and annoyed and your annoyance is soon going to turn into anger. Your anger is scary, but I know that I can take it if it means making you understand that we are in danger. What if it wasn't a dream? What if it was a warning? What if I do nothing and then something awful happens? I need to make you understand that everything is not okay. Then there is screaming and shouting and running around the house, but it is you and me, not the gorillas. Back and forth between our bedrooms. So much shouting. I am shouting at you to realize that we are not safe, and you are shouting back at me that I need to stop shouting because I will wake up my sisters.

I feel a sharp pain across my cheek and I am not shouting any more. You have slapped me. I run into my room and bury my crying face in my pillow. I have a metallic taste in my mouth and I look at my pillow. My nose is bleeding. You have given me a bleeding nose. You are standing in the doorway. The marks the gorilla made are still there. You take me to the bathroom and clean my face. You sleep in my room.

The next morning, you tell me that my new punishment is that I will have to sit in the spare room for the amount of time I kept you up the night before. I am not allowed anything to distract me, no books, I just have to think about what happened. Last night we were up for two hours. So today I sit in the spare room for two hours. I have a piece of paper and a pen, so I write you another apology note. Of course I am so sorry. In the light of day, it is clear that there are no gorillas coming and we are safe. I feel sick with guilt and regret. I had so badly wanted to fall asleep and wake up this morning in my own bed. I wanted to have a nice morning and you to be happy with me. I wanted you to see how far I have come in the year I've been at boarding school. I write that I understand it was my fault that you slapped me, and that you were only trying to help me.

*

Sunday nights are difficult; I always want to go home with you instead of back to school. I think that it is made worse by the fact that you don't want me to come back with you at all. I think that a mum should be sad that her 11-year-old daughter doesn't live with her, but you aren't. You are relieved. You don't tell me this, but I know, I can see it. You walk on eggshells and hold your breath so that we can have a nice 24 hours once a week, but I can see you breathe out a long sigh of relief when you drop me back at the boarding house.

The headmaster's wife takes me under her wing. She makes brownies with me in her kitchen so that I have something to take in when it is my turn to bring cake to our tutor session. My math teacher shows me how to use my controlling brain to get obsessively stuck into algebra questions instead of scary thoughts. I still struggle with the girls in my year. I don't want to be as weird as I am. I want to find conversation easy. I don't want to be standing silently on the edge of the circle, only coming up with the right thing to say seconds after the conversation has moved on. But mostly I can handle the daytime.

There are now five hockey sticks in my bed. I try to wrap them up in my blanket, but they are difficult to hide. The housemistress calls me in to her office and I try to explain. As I say the words, I know that I sound crazy. This is not rational. This is not rational. I need those hockey sticks, and four isn't enough any more.

*

The headmaster's wife has asked me to be in a promotional video for the school. A camera crew will follow me around for a few days and interview me. I feel so honoured. I have always been such a mess, but now I get top grades and they want me to represent the school. They end up regretting that decision.

SLOW YOU DOWN

We splice our lives between two places for three years. Every Friday afternoon, I bundle your effervescent sisters into the car with a picnic and we make a mad dash in the bus lane till 4 p.m. Then we crawl along with everyone else to the motorway. On Saturdays, either your dad or I drive to the coast, collect you and drive back to the barn. On Sundays, we drive the 45 minutes back to the coast, singing all the way to put off the growing unease you feel about being dropped back, and then I drive back to the barn, pack up, put your sisters, warm in their pyjamas, in the car, and your dad drives the two-and-a-half hours back to London. I like that journey. All I have to do is sit and chat to your dad while the girls watch the same Barbie mermaid movie on a loop. Just as we turn into our street, your sisters miraculously fall into a deep sleep, thus ensuring they are carried upstairs to bed. For three years, they keep this brilliant back-breaking act up. It is all worth it for those happy, precious Saturdays, and feeling for one day of the week as if I have a functioning family.

Of course, there are moments when things go wrong, and you are physically too far away for me to help. You've entered a school with a pre-existing pecking order and few are prepared to budge up and make room for you. I pack you off with a "period" pouch with what you might need, just in case. It travels with you. One Sunday evening, you realize you've left it behind at home and you call me, upset.

"Don't worry," I tell you on the phone. "You won't start your period this week …" I mean, what are the chances?

You start your period. I am in the car with your dad when I get the phone call and I know as soon as you realize that you're on speaker and your voice changes, what has happened. I call you back. These are the moments I wish I would teleport myself back to you. Instead, I call the member of staff in charge. She is amazing with you, she's done this a thousand times before, she gets a couple of the older girls to come and talk to you and it is all handled brilliantly over hot chocolate and toast. I feel we co-parent with the school, and when things get tough, the headmaster's wife takes you under her wing and gently breathes confidence back in to you. When you left the school after three relatively happy years, I thanked the house staff and her for giving me my daughter back, as that is what I truly believed they did.

Perhaps it is inevitable that the more time we spend in the country, the less London appeals. Your sisters start to envy your version of life. Frankly, so do your dad and I. The road signs around your school say SLOW YOU DOWN and eventually, we decide that is what we want for our whole family. Three years after you leave London, we follow suit. We want to be near the sea and under stars, the girls want a dog, and the move would mean we are all living under one roof. As we should be.

"You guys don't work so well as a five," my friend reminds me. She is worried that without your special status as the weekly returning prodigal child, the fight for attention will begin again.

"Surely we're beyond all that?" I reply, dismissing her concerns but feeling a little bruised by them – does she think I can't manage my family? What if she's right? Why is it so hard for us? … I push the feeling of inadequacy away. We have made up our minds. We want to extend our children's childhoods; I see too many 12-year-olds with handbags shopping in Westfield and wearing make-up, and it looks alarmingly precocious to me. Plus, we want our weekends back – the Friday–Sunday slog is taking its toll. I believe we can have a different sort of adventure outside London, so we follow our trailblazing eldest and, when the school year ends, we move to the country.

*

It is now September. Your sisters, aged nine and eight, go bouncing into their new school. They slip easily into the place they'd been visiting for three years. You head off to senior school, finally a teenager, looking so grown-up, beautiful and confident. I am filled with joy, everyone is happy, we are ready to meet new people and start to build a life.

We have found an old farmhouse to rent just 15 minutes from the school, and we move in. I am excited about being in one place for a while, and set about making it feel homely. It is a long, thin house, but redeemed by an Aga-warmed pale blue kitchen with a central island, a farmhouse table, a small fireplace and an old sofa to collapse into in a big bay window looking out over endless fields. There are working fireplaces in every room, which I look forward to lighting when the days darken. It is hard to imagine the cold since the sun seems to shine all the time. We are loving the salty-kisses, sandy-toes, rural-idyll life. We have tea on the beach after school, swim in the sea, watch the sun go down. Everyone says hello in this little Georgian town. I feel smug, smug, smug. Honestly, for three weeks, it is perfect.

Part 2

I'M NOT READY FOR THIS

It is my first day of upper school. I am 13. Most kids from my last school continue to this one, but there are still lots of new people, new teachers. A fresh start. I don't know what to wear to the welcome day. We are allowed to wear our own clothes today instead of the school uniform, which is terrifying. There have been times over the past three years at boarding school where I've decided, "Fuck everyone else, I am just going to be myself and wear what I want." This usually lasts a day, and then the sniggers, comments and looks become too painful, so I quietly slip back in line.

At my new school, I can't decide if I want to be invisible or if I want everyone to notice me. I can't decide if I want to be original or if I want to blend in. Who am I kidding? I am not brave enough to be even vaguely original. I would rather cover up my quirks and get through the next five years peacefully. I've always stood out a bit. At primary school, I went to the home-clothes day wearing my underwear over my leggings so that I looked like a superhero. I told everyone that I was the superhero who was going to stop bullying. I also had crazy red frizzy hair and a fuzzy fringe that my granny had cut for me.

Probably the most embarrassing thing I have ever done was in year 5 at my primary school in London. During Mr Carter's English class, I went up to his desk to show him my work, but I had to wait behind a girl who was already speaking with him. I stood there bored, watching everyone else scribble and stare down at their books. With my hands in my dress pocket, I wondered how low could I manoeuvre my pants down before they completely dropped to my ankles. I fiddled with the waistband until my underwear was somewhere near my knees. Oops. They fell to my ankles, and as I quickly dropped down to get them back, I hear Mr Carter's booming voice saying, "Right, class", and everybody looked to the front of the room – to me. I yanked my pants back on and my dress blew up like Marilyn Monroe's. I don't know how I ever showed my face at that school again.

Today is a fresh start at senior school, a whole load of new people who don't know the weird girl I used to be. Today is not the day to stick my head up above the parapet.

Keep your head down, Roxy.

Today, I need to find the right people and make them like me. I don't want to be mean – I am not a mean person, but on this battlefield, it is every woman for herself. And this time, I am not going to be shot down for trying to help the little guys. When I was 10, on the first day of boarding school some people were throwing a tennis ball at a boy over and over again in the corridor. I, not knowing any better, told them to stop because they were hurting him. They looked at each other, smiled, and started throwing the tennis balls at me. Not this time.

I put on a pair of black skinny jeans, a navy sweatshirt and my new Adidas Superstars – my first cool pair of shoes. I stand in front of the mirror with a face of disgust. The black and blue merge together so that I look like one big ball of dullness, like tar. I might as well just melt away because there is absolutely nothing individual about me. I want to be interesting and wear outrageous clothes and look different, but I don't have what it takes. I think that I used to have that sort of courage, but over the years, it has been chipped away, and now I am left with just enough bravery to get myself to school. The only thing that stands out is the white Slazenger panther just above my left boob. I whisper to the panther, "This isn't me, I promise." I slide my fingers through my newly straightened hair – nobody will know that I actually have a lion's curly mane. On my way out of the house, I grab my red bandana and tie it around my head, allowing myself one piece of the old me.

In the car, I practise conversation starters in my head. I remind myself how to sound like I'm not nervous and I don't give a shit about what anyone else thinks of me, when in reality I am terrified and all I can think about is what everyone else is thinking about me. "Just be kind, everyone will love you" are your words of wisdom. You have no idea – kindness gets you nowhere. As I walk towards the building, I chicken out at the last minute, yanking the bandana off my head and stuffing it in my pocket.

Be cool.

But I am not cool. I laugh at the geeky girl's joke and then instantly regret it – everyone stares at me. It turns out that the cool people's conversations consist only of bitching about other girls. They don't like me, I can tell. They can see through my shield of navy and black. They can see that I am weird. Afraid. I try to be funny, but it isn't the normal kind of funny. Here, being rude and mean is funny.

My pink Nokia brick, which bounced when dropped out of a second-storey window, has been upgraded to a sparkling iPhone. We all sit there aimlessly scrolling through pointless images and pretending to talk to our hundreds of friends. It beats making eye contact and having awkward conversation. I don't have anybody to text apart from my parents and I have nothing to scroll through on Instagram, so I slide repeatedly between the 10 photos I have on my phone of my granny and my dog. It is easier for everybody to pretend they have an exciting social life going on behind their screen than to make an effort with the people actually in the room. I am going to spend the next five years with these people and nobody is speaking.

One girl shows the two other girls something on her phone, they all start laughing.

Finally, I think, *some interaction*.

"What are you laughing at?"

"Nothing," they say in unison, and stop laughing.

I get through the first week by keeping my head down. I make sure that I am never seen walking alone. I cling to groups of people in the hour before lunch so that I don't have to sit by myself. It quickly becomes clear that my mission has failed; the right people don't like me and don't want to spend time with me. In fact, they cut up my sports kit so it is unwearable. They pour my new perfume on to my toothbrush and then fill it up with water. They hide my school uniform so that I am late to assembly.

I have never found school particularly easy. I can't say that it isn't my fault. I am the common factor, so it can't be a coincidence. I clearly attract it. The other challenge is that I am living at home for the first time in three years. I barely know my little sisters, as I went to boarding school when the youngest was only four. They certainly don't know me. You know me, though, and I get the feeling that I'm not someone you particularly like. I am nervous about living with you again, and I'm sure you are too. It has never been easy. I want you to like me, and I want my sisters to like me. I want to be mature and helpful and not cause any trouble any more. I know that I caused nothing but trouble last time, but I have changed, I promise. I've taught myself how to sleep on my own and not get so scared. I don't sleep with hockey sticks in my bed any more. This time, I am going to be easy and fun and we are all going to be happy. This is our new life.

*

Despite my reservations about my new school, I have a boyfriend. This helps me fit in. I am sitting on the sofa at my boyfriend's house and we are kissing. He is sweet. His name is Joe. He is very nice and we have absolutely nothing in common, but he really likes me, and I like being liked. Maybe it is because he is jealous that I am starting to get attention from older boys, maybe it is because he thinks that I am bored – either way, despite the fact that it took weeks before we even had our first kiss, he decides today that he wants to go a lot further, a lot quicker. He moves his hand down my waist, under my dress and tries to put his hand into my underwear. I push him away and jump up. I really don't want him to do that.

Luckily, 20 minutes earlier, I had started my period and am obviously way too scared to ask my boyfriend's mum for a pad, so I had stuffed toilet paper into my underwear. I therefore have the motivation of avoiding total humiliation to get me to push him away. I worry that without the bloody toilet paper in my pants, the fact that I didn't want it to happen wouldn't have been enough to make me stop him. I am 13 and confused. I didn't think that I would have to worry about these kinds of things for a while. A kiss is still a big deal to me.

SCHOOL GATE REQUIEM

The younger two have been tucked into bed; I still read to the seven-year-old, the nine-year-old reads to me. Bedtimes are now something I look forward to. Afterwards I go downstairs. You and I have found a programme to watch together every evening. I feel like I have a grown-up companion these days. It's nice, and I love it. You are finally the teenager you have for so long felt you are. Thirteen, my first real teenager. You have a grown-up bedroom just across the hallway from ours, with a dressing table and a desk. All is well. I glance at my phone. There is a text from my sister. I speed read.

... *the girls ... a tragedy ...*

My brain tries to put the information together but my heart is already sinking.

What? No, no. No. I must have made a noise, and you ask me what's wrong.

I don't know. The thing is I do know, I instinctively know. I call my sister. No answer. I call another cousin. I can't breathe. She tells me what she knows, which isn't much except that my cousin – a beloved, eccentric, fun, generous father of two and husband to a beloved wife – is gone. I slump to the floor and wail. It is telling that the little ones don't come downstairs even though they hear me. Years later, Ruby tells me she was trying to protect her little sister by saying it was just you and me fighting, and it is telling that Reva so easily believed her. How many blood-curdling rows, how much screaming, there had to have been in the past to make it a plausible excuse for the sound that came out from the pit of my soul.

I don't phone your dad; he is away auditioning and I know he'd hate to hear this terrible news so far from home. In the morning, I explain away the scream by telling your sisters I burned myself on the Aga.

Life is not the same after that. Joy is replaced by abject grief. I am a long way from home and I have no friends in this new place. But I do have purpose. I promise my cousin's wife she is supported by an army. An army we become, and an army we remain. She is absorbed into my life as a sister, her children become my nieces, and together, we co-parent through the bleakest of times.

There is a makeshift dormitory in my bedroom. Three mattresses side by side on the floor. The third is not for you; you sleep in my bed, the place you'd fought so hard to occupy, the place I'd defended with all my might. The third mattress is for my cousin's oldest daughter. She stays with us throughout the year, as often as she wants to and whenever she needs. She is seven. Although it sounds utterly miserable, it isn't always. We are a farmhouse of girls, often sitting around the kitchen table eating endless fish pies, you providing laughter and respite from the grief in the form of ridiculous year 9 gossip. A welcome diversion.

"So, any hot boys?"

"Who is getting with who?"

You chat hockey tactics and gossip with your little cousin, giving her a big sister that your own sisters probably envy. You are invaluable to me and to them and win yourself a place at the adult table. You've had your eye on it since you were four, but now you have earned the right to be here. Still, that doesn't make you a grown-up. One evening, you tell me a boy put his hand up your shirt. I am on the sofa, sewing name tapes into clothing. You've mentioned this boy before. He's a big guy compared to all the prepubescent lads in your year, and from what you've told me, he spells trouble.

"What did you do?"

"Stood up and ran away."

I can't remember if I suggested telling a teacher. It is possible I didn't, because whenever there are problems with your classmates, you never want to tell. You always say the same thing: "It will just make it worse." I say that means things won't change. It is an impasse I have arrived at with all three of you over the years.

"Are you okay?" I ask.

I can't remember your response.

A couple of weeks later, you announce that you don't want to go on the French trip to see the First World War graves. I feel like this is a backwards step.

"You should go. It will be fun, and you need to bond with your year group at your new school."

"I want to go to the funeral."

"No children are coming to the funeral."

You are furious. I know that look. You do not think of yourself as a child. You have been helping me look after the children.

"I don't want to visit graves."

Fair enough, all things considered, but still, I am a bit suspicious. You didn't want to go to the school trip to York when you were nine. I had to manhandle you on to the bus. You had to sit with a teacher. In the end, you had fun, but it was hell getting you to go. At 11, the only way to get you on the trip that term was to take you myself. Now that you're 13, I don't have the energy to manhandle you on to the bus and I can't take you to France, but you have to understand, stay or go, you cannot come to the funeral. Not even my cousin's children will be there. You want me to ask his widow to make an exception. You ask me this because you are not mature enough yet to understand how inappropriate that request is. I know you have seen a lot, but you don't understand as much as you think you do. I will not bother her with this, and I am not getting into a fight with you about my cousin's funeral. You're not going.

You go to the funeral.

The battle between us has been a long one. What you want versus what you need. It is not my job to give you everything you want; it is my job to make sure you get what you need. The funeral was a perfect example of the tussle between independence and dependence. You should not have gone, but I did not have the strength to fight on all fronts that day. I should have stood firm, but you are relentless, going on and on. I rolled over. I relented. It was a mistake.

SO MUCH FOR "SLOW YOU DOWN"

And then we get that awful phone call. I can't tell anyone what has happened; this is a small county, and gossip spreads like wildfire. I walk around school in a daze. That weekend, the whole family gather, people fly in. It's a quick hurricane of a weekend, and then everyone goes home again, leaving all the wreckage of the storm. The only people left are his kids, his wife and us. It isn't my loss or my grief, but the proximity to such a tragic death is doing something to me. I can't tell you how guilty I feel even saying that. I am so lucky. I just feel older now.

You are amazing. You scoop them up, you scoop us all up. His eldest daughter stays with us two nights a week. We all sleep in your room. You and me in the bed, my sisters and our cousin on three mattresses side by side on the floor. The farmhouse you rented when we moved to the countryside is haunting. It is dark and cold – there is no heating; broken lightbulbs hang from the ceiling. It used to be a bed and breakfast, and the bedrooms down the corridor have peeling floral wallpaper. I have spent years teaching myself how to sleep alone, in the dark, without hockey sticks, and now here I am again. None of us are ready to go back to our own rooms. So we eat too much frozen fish pie in our dark, cold kitchen. We form a kind of girl army. Dad is working a lot, but when he is home, it feels kinda wrong. He sleeps at the other end of the house. Even the word "Daddy" feels loaded and makes me tense up when my cousin sleeps over. It's like we can't really let him in. Us seven girls stick together. We talk about who likes who and who's kissing who. We create a new normal.

*

The funeral is next week and I am supposed to be going on a school trip. I don't know if I can walk through the graves of the First World War while my whole family gathers for the burial.

I am sitting on the school field, feeling older and more mature than I am. Being faced with death has exhausted me but it has also given me the courage to be a little more like my true self. I am wearing my bandana and these huge colourful trousers made of patches. I am actually beginning to feel happy again; I am with funny people and it feels natural and normal. It feels nice that we are laughing. Then I feel guilty for feeling happy. I go to hug my friend Zane goodbye, and as I do, he whispers in my ear.

"If you do not let me touch your bum, then I will beat up your boyfriend."

I start to laugh, this is clearly a joke, but he hugs a little tighter until I am silent. Then he slowly moves his hand down on to my bum, squeezes, and walks away.

He looks back at me and his eyes are telling me that this isn't a joke, and it isn't over.

He is a big guy. I am angry that a big guy can make me lose control of my body with one sentence. I am scared because there is no doubt that he could hurt Joe if he wanted to, or me for that matter. I am a bad person because there is also this creeping feeling of excitement. This tingle of danger and attention. Then there is this guilty pride I feel because he wants me.

The next day, he wants a kiss.

*

I go to the funeral.

I should not be there.

I am in no way prepared for the raw outpouring of grief.

I wake up the next day to 15 missed calls from Joe and a voice message. Zane has cut him all down his arm with a knife. Shit. I did not think that he would actually do it. I told nobody.

It had only been a couple of weeks but already Zane's threats had escalated to "If you do not give me a blow job, then I will hurt Joe really badly." When he said that, I started to laugh, but he did not even smile, he just stared right into me. I am scared – that tiny bit of excitement and pride disappeared. I am really good at flirting but I have only ever gone as far as kissing a guy – anything more terrifies me. People sometimes call me a slut, and maybe I make them believe that – I am very good at pretending that I am much more experienced and grown-up than I actually am. So I said no and walked away. I thought that was it – the funeral has been so intense that I pretty much forgot about Zane. I told nobody about his threat. There was no way that I could talk to a teacher about this kind of stuff. I feel disgusting. They would've looked at me like I was disgusting. Zane then probably wouldn't have been punished because it was my word against his with zero proof. Then two days later we would've been back in lessons together with him making my life a living hell because I snitched. Now he has actually hurt Joe, and it is my fault. I said no, and that wasn't allowed. I was just a thing that he couldn't have, and that made him angry.

A week later, I am sitting in the kitchen doing homework. I haven't told you about Zane attacking Joe. With everything going on, it seems ridiculous to even give airtime to such an unimportant event. But it does feel important to me, and I feel so disgusting and dirty because of it. I am worried that you will be angry.

I tell you what has happened and your response is so much worse than anger. You don't even look up from what you are doing. What I have said is completely pointless information to you. You imply that it isn't the drama that I am making it out to be, you don't ask if I am okay, and we don't speak about it again. This situation with Zane is the first time that I have been made to feel like a thing, and I feel responsible. I hate myself for saying this, but part of me enjoyed it, almost encouraged it. I am angry at myself for coming to you. I should know better than to come to you looking for care.

*

I am now on a school trip. Zane has been expelled and I blocked him on all social media so he couldn't threaten me again. A friend posts a photo of us both on her story. Immediately a message pops up on her screen.

Tell Roxy I am going to kill her.

IN THE BLEAK MIDWINTER

"You scumbag!"

The youngest cousins shout out the best line from 'Fairytale of New York' by The Pogues in a show entirely orchestrated by you. You play the guitar and sing. There are jokes and dancing. We then cut nativity scenes out of blocks of cheddar in a race to make Baby Cheesus. I look around the room. Smiling, happy faces glow in candlelight, around a table scattered with Christmas detritus. We are having fun. It's a bloody miracle. You are pivotal in making Christmas a success, and I am proud of you. But when the celebrations are over, the decorations put away, the darkness and the cold take their toll. Winter is interminable. We have no neighbours and a pint of milk is 20 minutes away. I have to gather every ounce of energy to get out of bed and put on a brave face as the shock of my cousin's death continues to ricochet around our lives.

I know you are worried about me because one morning, after the school tragically lost a pupil to suicide, you recommend I go and see the counsellor who has been helping the students process grief. You think I am depressed. But I'm not. I'm sad. I am sad that he died. I am sad for his daughters. I am sad I will never get into any more crazy scrapes with my mad Russian-speaking cousin, but mostly I am alone. The counsellor's card sits on the mantelpiece. I don't make an appointment, but you are right about one thing: I need to talk to someone. The trouble is, I have no friends here. I didn't have long enough to make any before my cousin died and now I have no energy to make them.

Instead, I spend hours on the phone to another cousin, getting advice and insight from her on the tragic, traumatic loss of her mother, who died suddenly and terribly when we were 10. The last time I saw her, she gave me three wooden angels. They still sit on a shelf in my bedroom. I spent many weekends at her house, reading stacks of *Beano*s and eating unlimited ice cream. At her house, we were allowed anything.

I also talk for hours with my oldest friend in London. She knows what it is like to rebuild a life around a missing mast because her mother died after a heroic battle with an eight-year illness when we were thirteen. I can remember her coming into school the day after her mother died and sitting on my desk. I can feel my arm around her scratchy grey blazer. I remember telling her, rather bossily, that it had been two weeks and it was probably time to get over it. It is a miracle we are still friends. What was I thinking? I was a moronic 13-year-old who wanted her friend back, who would put tights on her head and sing Crystal Gayle songs. I know now that deep grief is not something you get over but rather something you learn to live around.

"After Mummy died, there were lots of people around," my friend says now, "all saying they would always be there for us then slowly, one by one, they disappeared. In some ways, that was worse than the first loss. Don't make promises to his daughters that you can't keep," she warns me.

I heed that warning, because she is right. The wider family seep back into their lives, but we remain very much on the front line. I try to be supportive while also parenting my own discombobulated children. I am simultaneously impressed by how all three of you manage to sit for so long in the proximity of death and traumatic loss, but equally aware it is starting to take its toll, not least on me.

I know I am spread too thin because I had been halfway through reframing photos and posters for the farmhouse with a box of charity-shop frames when my cousin died. By February, the masking tape is still halfway round one of them. It lies there, accusingly. I have retreated before even making it out of the gate. I've got to finish that job. Make this house a home. I don't. I have to save my energy for the big stuff. That was another mistake. Making the house a home *was* the big stuff.

MAXIMIZE YOUR ASSETS

"You cannot come into the cafeteria wearing that."

I am staying late at school tonight for a play rehearsal. I am in the queue for dinner when the male deputy head comes up to me and says this.

"The leggings are inappropriate, and you will not be served food unless you go and put some tracksuit bottoms and a jumper on."

I assume he is joking. I am wearing a baggy T-shirt and leggings. The only skin showing is my ankles and my lower arms.

As we are having this conversation, two boys walk in wearing shorts and a vest. So Mr Deputy Head thinks that I will distract the boys, or perhaps I might distract him. I think that we can give teenage boys slightly more credit. It isn't like they are going to stop eating their spaghetti, drop their pants and start wanking in the lunch hall because I am wearing leggings. You know what? I take that back. At this point, it wouldn't even surprise me.

I skip dinner and walk to rehearsal with a male friend. It's January, so it's pitch-black. A guy in the year above comes up to me and asks my friend if he has a torch. He uses the torch to look me up and down.

"Everyone is saying that you are really hot. I can see why people would think that."

Then he looks to the guy next to me and says, "Get in there!" and walks off. I feel so proud of his approval and I didn't even have to say a thing.

*

I'm at another rehearsal for the school play. I have always loved the theatre, but now I am standing way back swaying from side to side and mouthing the words of the song. It's not cool to be keen. I have just been making out behind one of the buildings with a guy. Joe and I aren't seeing each other anymore, he probably hasn't forgiven me for not reporting Zane's threat to a teacher before they went on the school trip. Anyway, this guy had put his hands into my back pockets when we were making out, and it felt weird having hands there. In fact, now, as I sway at the back of the stage, I have to keep turning around to check that nobody is touching my bum. It is like his hands have left some sort of mark on me because I swear that I can still feel them in my pockets.

*

A week later, I am in London with an old family friend, Alex. I get a Snapchat from an older guy from my school who has been texting me. It is a dick pic that I haven't asked for. Alex bursts out in snorting laughter –"IT LOOKS JUST LIKE A HORSERADISH!" So Horseradish becomes his nickname. We want to go shopping today but we have no money, so she goes into her parents' safe to try and find some. It is exciting. We roll around on the floor taking photos of ourselves and the stuff we found in the safe and send them to some of the boys that we have been texting. I mean how adult are we? We dress up in eight-inch heels, tiny shorts, unbuttoned shirts. Then we put red lipstick and mascara on and take photos of ourselves in the mirror. Then we put on push-up bikinis and pretend to take a shower, but just pose for photographs instead.

Alex tells me all her friends have sent photos to guys in their year at school and other schools too. When they have sleepovers, they put on Victoria's Secret push-up bras and take selfies. Alex met a guy from my school a couple months ago, and I find out that they have been texting every night since. She shows me videos he has sent her where the screen is black and he is saying, "Daddy's little girl, slut, you naughty girl" in the first one, "My dick and spunk all over you, all over your tits and bum" in the second one, and "I'm gonna bend you down and fuck you from behind" in the third one. Alex thinks this is the funniest thing in the whole world. I find it disturbing.

Today I also bought my first pack of thongs, a five-pack from Primark which cost £2.50. They are each a different colour –

blue, pink, yellow, green and black – and lacy. They are so uncomfortable, and they rub the top of my bum so it's red and sore, but they make me feel grown-up and like I'm not pretending so much.

Once I am home, Horseradish and I continue to text for a few weeks. At school, we don't speak, but on Snapchat, we have this whole relationship. He isn't very attractive or funny or kind – in fact, he is rude to me whenever we are in front of people at school. Yet I am flattered that he even wants to text me. I feel proud rather than insulted when I hear that he has started rumours about wanting to stick his tongue between the gap in my two front teeth.

At the same time, a guy three years above me texts me. Dan is good-looking and very popular. Everybody knows who he is. I don't pay him that much attention because I am texting Horseradish. Horseradish is the first guy to ask me for pictures. He asks every single night and I am bored of it. I have only ever sent him photos in a bikini or revealing tops and tonight I just cannot be bothered to send him anything. Saying no isn't really an option for me. If I say no, then he won't want to be with me or talk to me any more and I can't be alone. I look up "women in underwear" on Google Images. I find a photo that doesn't show the face and I send it to him in black and white. The girl in the photo has straight brown hair, but it is better than nothing.

That's not you.

It is me.

I turn off my phone.

Back at school, it seems that the more that older boys pay attention to me, the more the popular girls have time for me. It is strange, that. I'm not complaining, I could do with a bit of protection at the moment. I've always wanted to be liked and wanted. I feel like I am at the centre of it now, the centre of the conversations and the drama and the gossip.

Meanwhile, I am very worried about you. Winter is not fun in the countryside. The house is even colder and even darker. It's pitch-black when we leave for school in the morning and it's pitch-black when we get home. I hate the rain because I don't want people to know I have curly hair. You are struggling now. I get home late and we sit in the kitchen and you talk to me about death and selfishness. It's a lot. We don't even have frozen fish pie any more, it's cheese on toast and Heinz tomato soup. I try to tell Dad that I think you might be depressed. I tell him that there's never any food and he laughs it off. You have always hated food shopping, so you just don't do it. It feels different now, though. You seem different. The issue is that you always make a huge effort on Friday nights when Dad gets back from London. There is a pie in the oven and a jug of water on the laid table, so of course Dad thinks I am just being dramatic.

Also, I don't feel 13 any more. I don't think I look 13, either. Concealer hides my freckles and mascara means that my previously non-existent eyelashes can now flutter their way through anything. I have bigger boobs now – at least, the Primark "Maximise Your Assets" bra makes it seem so. I have a "nice bum". I am starting to get more attention; boys in the years above look at me when I walk into the room. The sentence "You're so fit" makes me glow with pride. I am aware of how tragic that sounds, but it's true.

GREEN SHOOTS

I am standing among a group of fast-talking women I don't know. The tennis coach has to resort to sergeant-major tactics to get them to listen. Everyone is laughing. I have forced myself to get out of my car and sign up. It's what I've been asking of the girls, and if they can do it, so can I. I will restart the life we promised ourselves when we left London. While the coach talks about footwork, one of the women subtly raises her arm, places it around my shoulder and squeezes. I don't look at her because if I do, I will cry. She knows. I don't know how she knows, but she knows. Afterwards, we go for a coffee and instantly become fast friends. Nothing like a crisis to cut through the small talk. She is one of the heroines of this story.

You gradually settle into the New Year. I notice small but significant changes in your personality. You stand a bit taller, smile more broadly. You pick up the positive and bring it home, telling me all about it. You begin to leave the negative where you found it. You chat team tactics with your dad; in fact all you have to do is say the word "Daddy" to remind yourself how lucky you are. You tell me about the friends you're making. You are invited to their houses on the weekends. I drop you off. I pick you up. I am delighted, absolutely delighted. This is a breakthrough for you, and I believe I know what it is: you have been pushed through the portal of life, felt death up close for the first time, and it has changed you. There is no going back, and you are kinder, more resilient and less self-orientated for it.

In my teens, I spent a lot of time in homes where there was an unfillable hole where a mother should have been. So I knew that, however irritating it was to be told to pick up wet towels and turn off lights and get off the phone and do my homework,

I was and remain bloody lucky to have my mum. Please God, long may that be the case. I believe that hating your mother is the single most ridiculous waste of emotional energy that adolescence ever invented. However evolutionarily crucial it is to leave the cave.

I am sitting on the floor of the old larder cupboard. It's where the BT router is and the only decent Wi-Fi in the farmhouse. It is freezing, but worth it to see my oldest friend's face.

"Your mum's death left an indelible mark on me," I say, FaceTiming her. "In a way, it made me who I am. Watching the girls now reminds me so much about back then. Not quite grown-up enough to be a grown-up but trying to make sense of it anyway."

"Not only will Roxy grow up, she will grow up better," says my friend.

I am so reassured by this. She has known you all your life, she has known how difficult it has been for you to get comfortable in your own skin. It was she who warned me when we all moved out of London that living under one roof was going to be a challenge. Despite my cousin's shocking death, we are happy. We are getting on well. We have a laugh.

"So much for the terrible teens," she says.

"Roxy became a teenager when she was 4," I laugh. "I think we are through the worst."

In the summer term, you get excellent grades and come first in the 100-metre race. The fastest girl in the year hasn't always been very nice to you, and you've tried many ways to overturn her attitude, but in the end, you earn her respect by beating her. You sit in a gaggle of girls, proud in your team athletic vests, talking PBs and starting positions, laughing and smiling. There is a party that night. Boys. Dancing. A sneaky beer. All is well. I look at the group and think I wish you knew how beautiful you all are.

Grab it, I think, *squeeze it, drain every drop. Life is precious. And short. Even when it isn't.*

"How's Rox?" asks another friend.

"Honestly," I reply, "she just gets better and better."

I'M NOT FRIGID

I can't really talk to you about anything. I guess we don't have that sort of relationship. Your whole vibe doesn't really scream "You can talk to me about anything, I really care!" It is slightly more sort-it-out-for-yourself, tough-love style, which is fine. You are icy cold. I respect it a lot, actually. I would much rather be tough as nails when I'm older than soft and sensitive. I *am* sensitive, though, and I guess I feel quite alone. I am slowly working things out for myself. What a blow job is, what sex really is, what boys are like. I am quite good at pretending that I am super experienced, but in reality, I've learnt most of what I know from listening to people's conversations. I pick up little things here and there and log them. That is how I learn to use a tampon later on, something I am terrified of. I may now look like a confident, slightly intimidating 13-going-on-16-year-old, but I feel like a terrified little girl just trying to keep up and get through. I am nervous to make out with guys, especially if they are a bit older, as I have absolutely no idea what I am doing. Literally not a clue.

I suppose I wish we had a slightly more open relationship, but I'll work it out. You get cross with me if you can even see my bra strap. I don't understand it. You say it sends the wrong sort of message. Personally, I don't see why wearing a bra is something to hide. Doesn't half the population wear one? When I spend time getting ready and doing my make-up, you tell me that nobody is going to be looking at me anyway. I know what you mean is that everybody will be so busy thinking about themselves that they won't have time to think about me. I know that you are not trying to insult me and yet it still feels like an attack, or just not what I need to hear at all. I would prefer a simple compliment. Then there is also the side of you that wants to be a little outrageous and edgy, who talks quite explicitly about sex over dinner. You are difficult to work out. You are a total feminist, except you are also traditional and backward.

*

I am finally the person who gets invited to parties. I am wearing black skinny jeans with rips in the knees and a grey cropped vest. Underneath, I am wearing my Primark "Maximise Your Assets" bra, which is rock solid, weighs a tonne and is three sizes too big for me. All the guys are wearing Hawaiian shirts unbuttoned all the way and the "edgy" girls are wearing bucket hats. At parties I had been to before, we had been allowed a glass of prosecco and then we had danced to *Grease* mash-ups; now there are bottles of vodka lying around and cigarettes everywhere. I am 13 and definitely the youngest here by a couple of years. I am terrified, but I am not going to let anybody know that; I am at a party, boys want to kiss me, and I have people running up to say hello and give me a hug. I don't drink anything – I know that I need to be completely with it for this, it's scary and I am so out of my comfort zone. The people staying the night are four girls in my year and about 20 boys in the year above, I spend the rest of the night with Horseradish making out and feeling each other up. I am so inexperienced. He puts his hand into my underwear. I make the noises I think that I am supposed to make, but I am definitely getting this wrong. I think that I am supposed to have shaved, but I have never done that before either. Jesus, I am such a joke.

When I wake up after two hours' sleep, he doesn't speak to me. He flirts with another girl in my year, he makes yet another girl breakfast and he won't make eye contact. Finally he tells me I look like shit. I think I am going to cry, so I start walking towards the bathroom. I have to walk through a group of guys sitting in a circle in the corridor to get to the toilet. "Excuse me," I say, and as I walk between them, one of the guys reaches up and pulls my tracksuit bottoms down. All the other guys burst out laughing and I laugh nervously with them, trying not to turn bright red as I yank my trousers back up and run. I slam the bathroom door behind me and burst into tears, sliding down the door until I am sitting in a ball on the floor. I was wearing a Victoria's Secret thong, but what if I hadn't been wearing anything? Why did they think that was okay?

I leave without saying goodbye to Horseradish, and I never message him again. My friend's dad drops me at my grandparents' house and I lie in bed hurt, embarrassed and exhausted. I hate Horseradish and I feel so unwanted – I can't stand it. I feel disgusting with nobody texting me, nobody wanting me. So I text Dan. It seems that I am only really worth something if boys are admiring me. I send Dan the first photo that day, in my grandfather's bathroom. I guess that is the start of everything going to shit.

*

The next morning, I wake up and feel dirty. I use the downstairs bathroom instead of the one I took the photo in last night. I wish I hadn't done it – but worse than that, I now have Dan's attention and I don't want to lose it. He guarantees my safety at school, he is better than Horseradish could ever be, but I am playing with fire. My intelligent, conscious brain fades while the insatiable fear of rejection takes over. I tell myself he likes me. He likes me so much he wants more photos. More explicit photos. The requests become demands and when I don't deliver...

Rox ur so frigid

The word "frigid" is an odd one. The definition is: "(especially of a woman) unable or unwilling to be sexually aroused and responsive". Synonyms for frigid include cold-hearted and uncaring. In the Urban Dictionary, frigid is defined as "An outdated, Victorian term used to describe women who aren't interested in sex. Only used today by drunk men in bars to explain why the woman they attempted to pick up wasn't interested." I prefer the second definition, but I hadn't looked it up on Urban Dictionary because I was a child of 13.

Despite the clear absurdity of the word, I am terrified of being called frigid. When Dan starts calling me frigid for not sending nudes, it genuinely hurts me. He has been asking a lot since that first photo I took in my grandad's mirror, but I've always come up with excuses that got me out of sending them and kept him interested: "I'm babysitting", "my sister is scared and is sleeping in my room" - anything.

He isn't buying it. Tonight, he says:

Rox ngl if you don't send any im gonna hav to tell ppl that ur super frigid

He's losing interest. He is going to tell everyone in his year that I am frigid, then it will spread around the school, then no guy will ever text me again. I will be completely alone - my friends won't want to spend time with me. Sending photos is pretty common; most people are doing it. If I say no, then why would he keep texting me if he can just text a different girl who will say yes?

So I arch my back to make my stomach seem flatter. I roll my knees in and a thigh gap appears, I cover my face in the mirror with my phone, take my top off and push my boobs together with my arms. I press the button.

Dan is typing...

Go on, take off the bra

I turn my phone off, bury myself in the duvet and cry myself to sleep, swearing that I will never do this again. I hate myself.

The "take off the bra" texts really confuse me. Boobs are so ugly, how could anyone get turned on by two lumps of flesh? Although all the guys said I looked much older, I had actually only got my period a year or so before, so my boobs were still unformed and slightly triangular – you know that prepubescent stage. My solution was to take my bra off and then cover my boobs with my arm – really sexy. Posing like this sometimes makes me feel powerful and strong, and sometimes it makes me feel small and stupid and vulnerable, and sometimes it is a mix of both.

Dan never texts me during the day, then at around 8 p.m.:

Rox, wat kinda mood u in

I'm busy

Silence for a few days. No texts. I see that he is active on social media and hate myself, wishing he would text me.

Rox, wanna have fun 2night?

Every text that I send back is well thought through, they have to be cool but not try-hard. I have to make sure they show that I'm not very interested while also ensuring that he definitely replies and stays interested.

Part 3

HELLO, BOYS

You will be turning 14 in July. Finally, you are catching up with your friends.

"What do you want for your birthday?"

"Hair straighteners."

"They will ruin your beautiful red curly—"

Eye roll.

I find a bra in the wash basket that stands up on its own. You buy a bikini that stands up on its own.

"If you were a brand," I ask, "what sort of brand would you want to be?" I've read *Untangled: Guiding Girls Through the Seven Transitions Into Adulthood* by Lisa Damour. I am trying to practise what I've learned.

Eye roll. If I open my mouth to speak, I get an eye roll.

Really? After everything we have been through you are really going to be that kid? We are incredibly lucky that my parents have let us take over their house in this county every summer since you were born, it's why we moved here in the first place. Growing up you were surrounded by cousins, biked for hours, built treehouses, explored. Now we have our own ancient Land Rover to pile into and drive overland for picnics and firepits and days on the beach. We have a puppy. It is a summer of freedom and well-earned fun, and yet something is not quite right. I see more of the pouty, selfie-obsessed girl and less of the bike for hours, climb a tree girl. Tensions are inexplicably rising.

A few of your new friends come over to celebrate your birthday. I'm afraid I am not so sure that I like them. There is too much attitude, too few manners, a great deal of hair flicking and always, always the bloody phones. They sit in circles and stare at their own screens.

Pout.

Click.

Pout.

Click.

Christ, I think, this is what you've coveted all these years.

"Can we have a beer?"

"You were only 13 yesterday."

"All my friends are about to turn 15."

This is true. You are a classic summer baby with autumn-baby friends. Just as you catch up with them, they pull away. You've spent your life playing rearguard action. So I relent. One Corona each, and the rest are a low-alcohol brand. Immediately, the phones come out. How many photos can one group of 14-year-olds take of themselves sucking on a bottle of beer? But hey, it's the "popular" girls at your "gathering", so I ignore my inner sergeant major and tell myself that you're happy. But I'm not sure that you are.

A few days later, a couple of other friends of yours send you a photo from a festival of a particularly handsome sixth-form boy. You are giggly when you gleefully show me the photo. This is the boy you've been talking to. By "talking", you mean texting. I try not to overreact, run screaming to Travis Perkins, buy many pallets of bricks and build a tower so tall … You get the picture. I give him a once-over. No doubt he is handsome, but what you see and I see are completely different. You tell me about his sullied reputation, you tell me that he'd allegedly got a girl pregnant, you tell me he is a bit of a druggie, and you tell me he keeps messaging you.

"But he's actually really nice …"

The bricks aren't going to be enough. I try and counter your enthusiasm by telling you he has classic bad-boy idiot written all over him. I tell you that when I was your age, my best friend loved bad boys and I had to watch from the sideline while she repeatedly got used and then kicked into touch. I tried to intervene, but she took it badly – did I not think she was good enough? Quite the opposite, I tried to tell her, I thought *they* weren't. Her retort was always the same.

"It's not my fault I like the bad boys …"

Really? I always wondered. *Then whose fault is it?*

"Don't be that girl," I say. "Be smarter than that."

I try and warn you as best I can and tell you what my mother told me that she'd been told by her mother when she was 18. In 1960, on the cusp of the sexual revolution:

"Be careful. Mud sticks."

You are not listening to me. I know that because you want to spend more time with your very beautiful, sophisticated London cousin, rather than your fall-off-a-chair, giggle-until-you-feelsick American cousin who is over for the summer.

One evening, we have a family BBQ – which, for our family, means up to 50 people, and that's only the ones who live nearby. At the end of dinner, you insist on going home with my mother, and I think you're slurring your words. I don't want you to go because you have not been particularly pleasant and I don't like rewarding poor behaviour.

"Why can't I go? What difference is it to you?"

"Are you drunk?"

"Are you mad?"

Your words don't come out right. You stumble. Mum and I look at each other.

"Christ, I only had one Corona."

I don't believe you. I hate not believing you; it makes the ground shift beneath my feet. It is true I had let them all have one, but one Corona does not make you rock like a Weeble. I don't like being played for a fool.

"It's fine, she can come home with me," says my mother, stepping in. No one wants a showdown between us, they've all witnessed too many bedtime dramas. Frankly, after hearing that insolent tone in your voice yet again, I am happy to see the back of you. I am so bored of constantly monitoring the phone, correcting the attitude, reminding you of your manners. You are happy to go. A bit too happy. What am I missing? I am missing something.

"Mum," I say, pulling her to one side, "make sure you turn the Wi-Fi off." I have a sneaking suspicion you like going there because of the unfettered access to the internet. In the police state that I enforce, you only have Wi-Fi in the kitchen.

The following day, you don't come home. Instead, you've somehow arranged for my mother to drive you to my great-aunt's house. I don't have eyes on you. I know that's bad, but since I don't like what I am seeing, I am content to look away. You stay for a few days to hang out with the sophisticated London cousin. You are drawn to her like a moth to a flame.

"I think you need to go and get Roxy," says my mother.

"Why?"

"Just go and get her."

I am holding a cup of tea while my kind-hearted great-aunt spits uncharacteristic venom and paces furiously around her newly painted farmhouse kitchen.

"It's disgusting. I mean, why do they do it?"

I ground my feet. My mother has warned me that my great-aunt is losing her patience and wants the girls out of her house.

"They do nothing except take photos of each other. It's revolting."

She stares perplexed at me, genuinely upset, exclaiming, "I hate it, I hate it!"

"I know it looks bad."

"It *is* bad!"

I continue cautiously. "We don't get it, we don't, but things are different now. It's like their version of flirting—"

"They look like porn stars."

Bit harsh. Through my eyes, it was asinine, puerile nonsense and obviously really annoying, but through her eyes, it was something else, something awful, base and ugly.

"They are all doing it."

The explanation sounds thin because it is thin.

"But why?"

I couldn't answer that question. I try to talk to you on the way home, but you spit equal venom back. I don't want the fight and drop into the only safe place I know: silence. I really thought all this antagonism was behind us. It is boring, unnecessary and just ruins everything.

A couple of days later, my sisters sit me down and show me a picture you have posted on Facebook. It is you in that bloody padded bikini leaning up against a wall, your head thrown back, your bum pushed out, agent provocateur. My immediate reaction is jumbled. There is a jerk reaction of disapproval and concern accompanied by a bubble of pride. I try to focus on the positive. It isn't hard to see.

"She looks good."

I know as I hear the words emerge from my mouth that they are wrong, although you do. You look amazing. But through the concerned eyes of your aunts, looking good is not the point. Not the right point. On second viewing, it is clear this is too much exposure for a girl who has only just turned 14, overly sexualized, overtly sexy. I recognize the location with a sense of disquiet. It's my great-aunt's house. She had seen you take these photos and tried to warn me, but I could not imagine and failed to hear. I wait till I see you alone.

"Listen, that photo—"

You cut me off. "I've taken it down."

"Right. I mean, you looked stunning but it was a bit—"

"It's gone, it was stupid, it's gone."

I repeat the golden rules, the ones I have repeated and by the way, still repeat. My fail-safe litmus test.

"Don't post anything you wouldn't want your grandparents to see. What goes online stays online. FOREVER!"

You look at me as if I know nothing and of course, I know nothing. I am trespassing in your digital world, but the virtual world is lawless and it scares me, especially since it feels as if someone took my sheriff badge away.

You find my presence more disdainful than usual. Sometimes I don't even get a scowl, as if I am not there at all. You pretend not to see me or hear me; sometimes it is so obvious that it's funny. But mostly it isn't. It still isn't. It is rude. I have always struggled with your rudeness and I am depressed that it seems to be getting worse, I cannot bear to think we are returning to the bad old days of antagonism and fury. Something is going on, I realize that, something I can't grasp. You have only just turned fourteen, you're a child, despite what you think. I can see your head has been turned, my job is to stop you leaping into the flames. I don't mind being the bad guy but I don't want to be perpetually punished either, so I keep repeating the golden rules.

"Don't be that girl."

"Mud sticks."

"FOREVER!"

No wonder you didn't want to hear what came out of my mouth.

Summer begins and so there are hours to fill. I have no work to do, as I've decided that school isn't really very important in the grand scheme of things. We are spending the summer at the rented barn with lots of glass because it is near my granny's cottage. The attention becomes an addiction. If I haven't been told how "hot" I am that evening, I can't sleep. If I don't have five boys texting me at any one time, I stare at myself in the mirror and try to work out what is wrong with me.

For the first time in my life, I look forward to going to bed. Bed doesn't mean sleep any more. Bed means attention and flattery and time alone with my phone. Bed means that I get to feel good about myself.

It is my 14th birthday and I am so proud of myself. I have three friends over – they are popular and mean, but I like myself more now that I am their friend. We are allowed two beers each, so we take lots of photos posing with the bottles and posting them on social media. My friend from school sends me a photo from the festival she's at. The photo is of Dan and next to him is this really, really overweight guy. Dan looks amazing. Now every-body knows that I am texting the fittest guy in school and that gets me – I want to say respect, but it is more like the opposite. It is a backwards kind of respect where everyone knows that what's going on is fucked up, but it still means that they want to spend time with me.

"This boy is texting me, isn't he gorgeous?" I brag to you.

I am drinking alcohol, bitching about other girls in my year, posing for photos and Dan is texting me – I have made it. He sends me a text saying that we should "hav sum fun later". A tingle of excitement and fear rushes through my body. I probably won't text him later, but just knowing that he wants me to makes me glow. I make sure that the other girls know that I am texting him – I don't tell them directly, but I leave his name on my phone for them to see. I guess I am showing off. Later on, he texts me telling me to go to the bathroom, so I do. He tells me to undress down to my underwear, so I do. I am wearing one of my new thongs that I bought from Primark and have hidden from you. He tells me to take my bra off and prop my phone up, so I do. He tells me to get down on my hands and knees and arch my back slightly. I take the photo and I send it.

"I can't get my head around how every time you go into the bathroom you take all your clothes off, take a picture, put your clothes back on and just carry on with your day," my friend says.

They aren't mean to me about it. A few people say that it isn't very smart, but most people just laugh at it, and I tell myself that they are slightly impressed. Maybe they are, maybe they aren't, but they are at my house – which never would have happened six months ago. Everybody knows how good-looking Dan is, and I am proud that he wants me.

I have a present for you, Dan types.

He sends me a dick pic and starts typing out sexual texts, telling me to put my hand down into my underwear and finger myself. I pretend that I haven't read it, turn my phone off and go to sleep. I can't handle that.

*

I am at a family BBQ and I have a beer in my hand. I am looking out at the sunset, sticking my bum out and fake laughing with my sophisticated cousin from London while the camera clicks behind me. I am spending less time with my funny, clumsy, childish, loving, incredible cousin from New York. I do not tell her about the photographs, because she won't understand. I also don't tell her because I know she won't approve. I do not want to play in fields and have picnics on hay bales and pretend that everything is perfect. Everything is far from perfect. I am not perfect. I look at you smiling, laughing and eating cold sausages and I hate you for not seeing it. If only you knew how disgusting I really am. My cousin from London gets it. In fact, she encourages the photographs; she does it all the time. You look at me with the same boredom and anger in your eyes.

"Roxy, you are drunk."

I am not drunk.

I go to stay at my granny's house again. I still really struggle to sleep at the barn because those big black windows are still scary, it is still in the middle of nowhere and I still have memories from bad nights there when I was younger. The marks on the door from the gorillas are still there. The hours I spent in the spare room as punishment for the hell I had caused the night before. My sleep got better when I was 12, but since your cousin died, I have spent many more nights sleeping in your room. My granny's house feels safe. It also helps that when I am at her house, I don't have to look you in the eye. I feel like if you stare at me for long enough, then you will see through me – see how disgusting I am and the awful things that I am doing. It is best to avoid you.

The Wi-Fi turns off when I get into bed and I immediately know that my granny has unplugged it on your orders. I sneak down and turn it back on when I think she is asleep.

The following morning, completely understandably, she is cross.

"You cannot just do as you please in other people's houses."

She doesn't realize how painful it is for me to lie here and feel unwanted. Without Wi-Fi, I lie here and hate myself. I need the attention, but more importantly, the distraction. I cannot have time to think. Thinking kills me. I am trying to explain this feeling. This feeling that I am lying in bed, empty and pointless. That without a buzz I might die. I think that this might be what addiction feels like.

It feels like you are just scrambling around for ways to control me. I am so angry at you for picking and choosing which parts of parenting you want to do. You can control and punish, but you can't be there for me or help me. I make a promise to myself that if I have children, they will always know that I am on their side and that they can come to me, no matter what they have done. I will make sure they know that I am ready and open to having any conversation, even if it involves things that I don't understand.

I am angry at you for trying to damage my relationship with my granny. I feel safe here. And my grandad's bathroom has the perfect mirror for taking photographs.

*

My London cousin is showing me the collection of photographs of herself on her phone. She looks amazing. She has an app on her phone which looks like a normal calculator, but if you type in a specific number, then it takes you to this secret photo album. That is where she keeps her photos. We get changed into our bikinis and take photos of each other posing in different places around the pool. Obviously, we don't actually swim, because we have straightened our hair and we have a lot of make-up on. The picture I look best in is one of me in an archway. I am facing the side with my hands on the wall, my back arched so that my stomach is flat and my bum is sticking out. I am wearing a leopard-print bikini and I look good. I feel proud.

"Post it on Facebook."

I hesitate.

"Go onnnnn, you look so hot!"

Fuck, I don't know. I look good. Dan will like it, all the boys will like it and the girls will be jealous. It just feels wrong. As I click the "post" button, I feel like I do every time I send a photograph. A buzz of excitement because I am proud of how I look, and a creeping dread because I know I am screwing up. This is different to sending a photo to a boy, though, because everyone will be able to see this. I post it anyway, and immediately the comments and texts start to arrive.

FITTTTT

WOW OMG THIS IS GORGEOUS

SEXY 🔥

I am seriously glowing when I suddenly see that my aunt has liked it. Shit. This is wrong – everybody can see this. I feel so dirty. I take it down and I am sad, because having it up on Facebook made me feel good.

You try to talk to me about it. I don't want to talk to you. You don't understand. You are just so angry at me. I resent you for trying to have an honest, open conversation about this with me. You lost the right to do that when you made me feel that I could not come to you with these problems. You don't get to pick and choose. Either you are there for me with advice, help and a hug or you dismiss my cries for help as attention-seeking, but you don't get to do both; and you chose the latter a long time ago.

Another guy in sixth form at school starts texting me. His name is Ryan. We actually get on; he is smart and we have conversations. He never asks me for photos, but one night I send some anyway. The empty, pointless feeling is just too much and I cannot handle it. Nobody is texting me and I feel this deep pain inside: this invasive thought that the world is going on without me, outside this room, and it doesn't want me anywhere near it. I know that Ryan likes me and he finds me attractive, so I send the photos. It gives me that brief relief from the pain, but it doesn't last long enough. It never lasts long enough, and what's more, I have screwed it up with Ryan, who is a friend, nothing more.

I don't want you to think that sending photos means nothing to me. I feel disgusting all the time. I hate myself, I feel dirty and I don't want anyone to come near me in case they notice how disgusting I am. You think that I am pushing you away because I am rude, but actually, Mummy, I am just so ashamed.

NO HARM DONE

I am halfway through taking three daughters'-worth of toys and hand-me-downs to Oxfam when I get a phone call from the mother of the friend you are staying with.

"Roxy is arranging to meet some older boys at the beach. Sixth-formers. I thought you should know."

I wasn't sure how to respond. *Thanks?* I call you immediately. "Where are you?"

You tell me something hurried and not entirely convincing. I let it slide because what can I do? I am packing up our old house, 140 miles away in London, so I have to take your word for it. I want to take your word but I don't really take your word for it. Anyway, there is a bigger issue building on the horizon. A party.

"I don't know if I should go to the party ..."

Even I am nervous about this party. I've heard that parties at this household are unstructured, unsupervised and liberal with the alcohol, but getting to this party has taken military-style operational planning and you have impressively organized it all. Since I am away you will be dropped in a supermarket car park to wait for a friend, her dad will pick you both up and drive you to the party, which is 45 minutes away. The following day, another girl's mother will collect you and drop you at my parents' house, where you'll stay until I get there with the removal van. I have spoken to all the parents involved in your convoluted plans, except the woman who is actually hosting the party. It would take quite a lot to undo it all now, and anyway, where would you go if you didn't go to the party?

"You'll be fine. Just take care of yourself and don't drink."

"I'm nervous."

You are always nervous about parties. I call the mother hosting the party, so I know an adult is in charge. This way, you and I are both reassured.

"Sorry to bother you, just checking that you're expecting Roxy tonight. I'm calling because I am in London packing up the house –"

"Absolutely, of course. Don't worry, my daughter is really looking forward to seeing her."

"Great. Will someone be there to keep an eye? Thing is, she's only just 14 and I can't come and get her if there is a problem." I chicken out of saying: "Please don't let her drink herself into a stupor, and if she does and is sick, you are in charge and are legally responsible for her safety."

"That's fine, they're all staying the night. My elder children will be keeping an eye."

That is what I am worried about. So I press on.

"But will there be an adult there?"

"Absolutely, she'll be fine."

I feel the woman isn't really listening to me – she sounds distracted. I must sound like an overly anxious parent, one she'd like to get off the line, so I end the call.

Minutes later, you call again. I am expecting you to tell me you're in the car, but I can tell immediately that something is wrong. You are crying and trying to speak.

"I've been disinvited to the party."

"You can't have been, I've just spoken to the mother, and she said her daughter was looking forward to seeing you."

"I'm telling you, I'm not invited. I can't go. I don't know what to do."

"Stay there. I will call her back. They can't leave you stranded in a car park."

I am not too worried at this point. Surely, there must be an explanation. I call the mother back, certain that she wouldn't condone leaving a child stranded in a supermarket car park.

"I'm sorry to ring again, I've just received a call from –"

"Yes. Seems there was a misunderstanding."

"What? You just told me your daughter was looking forward to seeing her, that I had nothing to worry about."

"Yes, sorry, as I said, there was a misunderstanding."

"What misunderstanding?"

"She wasn't invited."

"She was. I saw the text myself. It has all been arranged. She is currently alone, waiting in the Tesco's car park, and I am in London. I can't go and get her."

"Not sure what happened."

"But you told me your daughter was looking forward to seeing her."

"I don't know what happened."

It doesn't seem to matter what I say, it doesn't seem to matter that you are dumped, stranded and alone, the woman does not care. I keep thinking she'll realize and say something else, but she chooses not to and it is unfathomable to me. While

I feel sick for you, I am grateful you will not set foot in this woman's house.

I ring my mother who kindly agrees to go back to the coast and get you. It is a two-hour round trip for her. She's 74. I ring the other mother who'd given me the heads up about the older boys and she offers to fetch you and lets you stay with her till my mother arrives. All this is done by frantic phone calls from an empty house in London between taking the curtains down and lugging them over to the dry cleaners and stuffing my old city life into binbags with a knot of pure fury on behalf of my child.

It is not a pleasant day.

Though you are beside yourself in the car park, when you're safely back with your grandmother and sisters you tell me you're a bit relieved not to be going. I don't know whether it is self-defence or emotional maturity, but I am proud of your ability to rationalize such poignant rejection. I am exhausted and furious and still have the rest of the house to pack up.

Poor, poor you, I think, *at least you are safe, and this stupid little girl can't hurt you any more.*

The summer continues. I detect that the wounds inflicted by being disinvited to the party have left a little scar tissue because, for a brief moment, there is an interlude in the hostilities between us. There is a new enemy on the horizon and for the first time this summer, it isn't me. Older boys still circle. Your friend Ryan offers his help with the furniture that has arrived from London.

"Is it okay if he bikes over?"

Beyond it being a little odd because he's a sixth-former, I haven't got a problem with that, and I can't move this stuff on my own. Five minutes later, you're back.

"Maybe he shouldn't come."

"Okay."

"You don't want him to come."

"I don't know him."

"I thought it would be helpful."

"It would be."

"So you want him to come."

"Either way is fine."

"So do you think he should come?"

Round and round.

When he does arrive, he is actually very sweet, a bit nerdy, good at maths like you and I can see why you like him. He is the opposite of a threatening bad boy, he is polite, shakes my hand, just about looks me in the eye, helps me move furniture and passes the audition with flying colours except there isn't a role on offer.

He asks you to his birthday party. Another roundabout debate. Should you or shouldn't you go? I even discuss it with my sisters. I constantly feel like I am pulling the reins of what you want versus what you need. Let's be honest, why would a kid not yet in fourth year go to a sixth-form party? It doesn't seem right, especially since it means missing your American cousin's last night in the UK, but you say you want to go. In the end, I call his mother. I am not making that mistake again.

The year difference is a bit pronounced, we agree.

But, she says, he is not hugely sophisticated – he is a gentle, rather naive young man.

She is very nice and assures me her son will look after you. We agree that forbidding you seems heavy-handed, and though I may be an authoritarian, forbidding isn't my style. Recently, educational psychologists have concluded that your average 14-year-old girl thinks like a 17-year-old and the average 14-year-old male thinks like a 12-year-old. You are older than your years. He is younger. Perhaps it isn't so odd.

You and I agree terms: I will take you. I will also pick you up a couple of hours later. No smoking. No drugs. One beer. You must be exactly where you say you will be at exactly the time you say you'll be there, not one second late. I am proud of you, you don't squeeze yourself into a backless-frontless-sideless dress, you wear flares and a jumper, a little make-up. Since some of the girls in your year continue to be foul to you after the previous party debacle, what is so wrong with getting a bit of protection from a handsome prefect maths geek?

When I pick you up, you tell me the bad boy is there, smoking dope by the bonfire. You tell me who is nice, who is not and who is surprised to see you there. You have a good time and I am pleased about that. You didn't even have the allocated beer. All in all, you are happy that you'd gone, and it had been a success. No harm done.

IMPLOSION

A text mentioning photos pops up on my phone. I reach over to turn the screen over, but it is too late, you have seen it. I really do think about telling you, in that moment, just to say that I have messed up. It's embarrassing, yes, but probably not the end of the world. I know that if I tell you, then I will never do it again. I almost crack and let it all come out. You look at me and there is so much dislike for me in your eyes. *My mum doesn't like me.* I don't tell you. I mumble some pathetic explanation for the text, glare at you, and then avoid eye contact. I do stop sending photos, though. Suddenly, the fragility of my situation is much clearer. I realize that I am no longer in control of what happens to me. With every photo that I have put in the hands of others, I have given away a slice of control.

Dan quickly gets bored of texting me now that I won't send him anything. At night, I see that Dan is active on social media and the fact that he doesn't want me any more causes me physical pain. It takes all my willpower to stop myself sending anything. I want to feel that buzz again. I feel hollow as I stare up at the ceiling, willing myself not to turn my phone back on. I think I know this feeling. I am hollow on the inside. Whatever I pour in drains away. I am always empty. A bottomless pit.

I feel completely worthless for days and days and then I start to feel better. I start to smile again. I start to leave my phone at home when I go for a bike ride and that feels okay. I start reading in bed again to keep me distracted. I start to enjoy where I am again and actually feel happy.

*

I am at my friend's house and I get a Facebook message from a guy I don't know, named Aiden.

Hey, I think that you are really fit.

I vaguely recognize him and his profile says that he goes to my school. I ignore his first few texts. His fourth text asks me to send him photos. I ignore again. The fifth text comes. It is a photo of me in the mirror in a bra and thong. It is clearly me. Taking photos like that became so normal for me that I had stopped scrubbing my face out. Idiot. I had sent some of them on Snapchat. Of course, Dan always promised not to screen-shot the photos, and Snapchat notifies you if your images have been screenshotted by whoever you send them to. But there is a separate app that lets you screenshot without the other person knowing, and anyone can take a photo of a photo. Shit. I feel sick. Then I realize why I recognize him: Aiden is the big guy who was next to Dan in the photo my friend sent me from the festival. And then the killer text. The one that marks the end of my childhood.

If you don't send me what I want, then I will send the photos I already have to my cousin.

His cousin is a girl in my year, Liz. She is very popular. She isn't that pretty, but she has big boobs and rich parents who let her have parties with no supervision, so everybody loves her. If she gets those photos, then everybody will have them and I think I might die. So I go to the bathroom and strip down to my underwear. I am wearing an M&S bra with big pants because I'm on my period. I take the photo and crop it to cut out my pants so that he doesn't see my pad. I feel small and weak, I am shaking. This isn't fun or exciting, this isn't what I want. I do not know this person, I've never met him or spoken to him and until a moment ago I didn't know his name, yet this big seventeen-year-old guy holds my life in his hands. I want him to leave me alone. I was in control before – I swear I was.

I find out later that this guy and Dan had played Top Trumps with my photos at the festival.

I know that you are probably screaming at me while you read this. I know that the more photos I send, the more ammunition he has. I know this, and yet I send them anyway. It is stupid and I am not thinking properly. The fear of everyone seeing these photos is controlling me – it has taken over the smart, rational part of my brain. I think deep down I know that I am making it worse by sending more photos, but I just cannot handle the alternative. The alternative is not an option.

I put my clothes back on and return to my friend's kitchen. I have a cup of tea and chat with her and her mum. I chat and smile with them and try to blink as little as possible. The second my eyes close, I see my body in the mirror. So I stare at a point until my eyes water. If Aiden sent the photos to Liz, then these people would see them. All my friends and their mums would see them. They wouldn't want me chatting around the kitchen table then. My friend wants to go swimming, but I tell her that I have my period.

"Just put a tampon in and let's go."

Shit. I haven't done that before. I know that this is the sort of the thing that I should just know how to do, I'm 14. Nobody showed me. I wanted to ask you a few months ago, but I was too embarrassed. I was at boarding school when I got my first period, so we never really talked about it.

She hands me a tampon and I take it into the bathroom. It is huge. What if I put it in the wrong hole? What if I don't put it in right and it falls out in the pool?

I feel around and just push it in as hard as I can. It hurts. This can't be right.

I walk out of the bathroom, holding my legs as close together as possible. I swear it isn't all the way in, it feels like it is slipping out.

I check my phone before I go outside, and there is a Facebook message from Aiden.

So fit.

He asks for more and more photos and his requests get worse and worse. I hate myself and I hate you for not being somebody I can turn to. I don't trust you not to be angry and I can't take anger right now; I need help. Every time I look at you, I hate you because you should be helping me and, instead, I have nobody.

*

I am sitting in the corner of my granny's spare room and I am crying. He has asked for a video of me fingering myself. How did I get here? I am smart. This isn't me; I can't have ended up in this situation. I want to die. I am completely stuck. Whether I send it or not, either way, I am fucked. There is literally no way out. I can't send the video. I can't cope with everyone seeing the photos. Why does my granny have such awful pink floral wallpaper? Salmon carpets, really? I bang the back of my head against the part of the windowsill that sticks out. I hate the pink and the flowers and the sun and the sheep in the field and the lace throw on the bed. I hate the mirror that is staring back at me, reminding me of everything that I have done. I hate you for not knowing. I hate my cousin for wanting to go on a bike ride. I hate my granny for asking if I want a cup of tea. I hate everybody because nobody can help me and I have absolutely nobody to blame but my stupid self. I eat some toast with Marmite and I hate it because I think I am going to throw up. I hate the mirrors.

I block Aiden on every social media and spend the next few days in a constant state of fear. Any second, everybody could find out what I have done, and they will see all the photos. You will see all the photos. I swear to myself that if the photos ever get out, I will kill myself. There isn't another option. I can't do this. I pray that Aiden is too embarrassed about texting someone so young to show the pictures to anybody. I pray. I think of Fatima and her stupid prayers and I recite them over and over and over again. I wish I had the fucking holy water right now. Draw a cross on my forehead please, I made a mistake – but Fatima said I could be forgiven.

*

Liz, Aiden's cousin, is having a party. We aren't very close, but the other girls going have become my friends. These are the girls who think that they are ridiculously cool because they sometimes smoke a cigarette and drink real alcohol. Anyway, I feel honoured to be invited. I think that the day I got the invite,

I began to like myself just a little more. You are in London, so I have come up with quite an elaborate plan to get myself to the party. My friend's mum is taking me to a car park to meet another friend, who will take me to the party. I also make a plan to meet Ryan at the beach before the party. When I wake up you call me and accuse me of meeting up with a bunch of much older boys without telling you. I try to explain that I am just meeting up with a friend, but you are stressed, so I drop it and tell Ryan not to come. I don't really understand how my plan managed to snake its way all the way to you in London in less than an hour, but that is what it is like living in the countryside. Everybody always finds out about everything. I am dropped at the meeting point and I sit on a low wall by the car park and wait. After about 15 minutes, I start to feel a low aching feeling crawl through my chest and down into my stomach. They aren't coming.

Eventually, I get a text from the girl who is supposed to be picking me up, saying that Liz has said that I am actually not invited to the party, so she has left without me. Since when did "Please come to my party" not count as an invite? This is humiliating. This is awful. I knew that Liz was not a good person, but these other people were meant to be my friends. I dig my knuckles into the corner of the brick wall I am sitting on. What if Aiden has sent her the photos? I am stuck in a car park an hour away from home, with nobody to call. You are in London. All my friends are at this party. What if Aiden has sent her the photos?

*

I find our enormous family difficult. It is very traditional and there is little room for individuality. You just have to shut up and get on with it, do what you're told and don't question anything.

There are too many kids, so no child is special and there is huge competition for attention. My granny has four siblings, you had sixteen first cousins and I have thirty-two second cousins and still counting. Some have relocated as far as Australia, some are just a mile away, but they all gather as often as they are able and it is chaos. You've never acted like you wanted us there. You were always complaining about us or trying to get us to leave you alone. So we did. We would scrounge together some food for a packed lunch and then go off on an adventure, not returning until the sun disappeared and our stomachs rumbled too loud to ignore. There were always too many kids to feed, so meals were small and simple. Four pieces of tortellini and half a sausage. I can hear your sarcastic tone now: "Yeah, you look malnourished. You poor, deprived child." We weren't poor or deprived or malnourished. We were hungry and a bit sick of constantly being sent away and made to feel like burdens. So we stole our grandfather's sugar cubes to suck on and occasionally a chocolate digestive, until he caught us one day and put a lock on the cupboard.

I feel like I am now beginning to see the cracks in this family. Before, our summer holidays seemed to have been lifted straight from an Enid Blyton novel, full of adventure and fun and freedom. Now it seems fake. I am beginning to notice the alcoholics who are "just stressed", and the anorexics who are "just on a health kick", and all the crazy that is unspoken about and covered up. If feelings always have to be kept inside, then of course people crack.

I have never been able to conform, in school or in our family. I have always been seen as the problem child because I wasn't good enough at hiding all my insecurities and my fear. I should have kept it all to myself like everybody else, but the fear was too much. Now, when I look around at the smiling faces of so many cousins, I just feel angry. Stop smiling! Not everything is perfect; bad things happen. Can somebody just acknowledge that not everything is perfect?

*

I spend my days between my granny's cottage and the barn, doing everything I can to avoid having to engage in a conversation with you. I pray some more and I hate myself more for thinking they wanted me at this party. I scroll through the photos they post, smiling faces posing with cigarettes that they don't know how to smoke. Aiden is in some of the photos, smiling like a creep at the back with these young girls who are wearing practically nothing. I pray some more. One day, I do go for a bike ride. I bike by myself to the farthest place I can think of. I walk through a forest area so I am surrounded by trees. I spin around as fast as I can until I feel sick. Then I fall to my knees and I scream. I scream until I cannot breathe, and I then I notice that I am on all fours, the same position I was in when I sent Dan that photo on my birthday. I stand up and scream some more. I am so angry at the world for letting this happen to me. Then my aggressive mind reminds me that I am the one who let this happen to me, so I shouldn't try to blame it on the universe. It doesn't occur to me to blame it on the boys.

The rejection from Liz's party has left a burning hole of self-loathing in my stomach. Now I am invited to another party, Ryan's birthday party. He is turning 18 and I have just turned 14. It is a bit odd. He is very sweet and nice and nerdy. I have been invited to a sixth-form party, so of course I am flattered. People already think I am a slut. It is just so nice to be invited, nobody else my age is invited. This battle between what is right and what makes me feel good about myself is exhausting and it is constant. I just want to be the person who gets invited to parties and who has fun and who people want to spend time with.

I go to the party. I wear baggy jeans, a jumper and just a tiny bit of mascara so that nobody can call me a slut. I let my hair be its frizzy, wild self for the night. I agree to your terms: no smoking, one beer, be in a certain place at a certain time. I can feel my aunts judging me as I get ready to leave the house. *I'm sorry that I am not as "good" as your daughters*, I think.

The girls at the party are nice to me, but they seem a little weirded out, which I get – it is weird that I am here. I don't understand why he wants to spend his party babysitting me rather than having fun with his friends. We walk past Dan and he pretends that he doesn't know me, gives me a hug and introduces himself. Fucker. I see Aiden and change direction. That man could ruin my life.

NO SUCH THING AS FICTION

You and I are sitting on a grassy knoll in the huge outdoor playground of a local nature reserve. The summer holidays are coming to a close, and this is the last mass family gathering before school starts. I am looking forward to school starting. It's time. I am tired of the backchat and bad moods.

This is a nice moment, I think, *please don't spoil it*.

"I've had an idea for a book," you say.

I should have shown more interest, but your venom had worn me down and I am carrying some scar tissue of my own. You want to chat, but I'm really not feeling the love.

"It's about a girl who's done the one thing that she's been told not to do and now doesn't know how to … tell."

I can't remember the exact words because I am only half listening while I unpack some sandwiches.

"Tell what?"

"What she's done."

"What has she done?"

"I told you. She's done something stupid …"

"What?"

"Doesn't matter."

"Give me an example."

"Like posting something on the internet, something she regrets."

"Like what?"

"Nudes."

I once tried to write a book about a protagonist who did something stupid and it was really hard to make the character likeable while watching her destroy her world. I rewrote the novel three times, so I know how hard it is. But what I am *really* thinking is if anyone is idiotic enough to post nude photos of themselves on the World Wide Web, then what the hell do they expect? I really need you to get this. I really need you to know how utterly stupid it is – the world is not kind to girls stupid enough to post naked pictures of themselves.

"It is such a stupid thing to do and it's hard to like a stupid character. They'd only have themselves to blame. I don't think it's a great idea for a book."

You stare daggers at me. Well, it's what I think, I know you're only a kid, but surely you must know this by now. You've been told a million times. That is the end of our semi-civil conversation.

I roll, oblivious, towards a new school year. One by one, the giant barrel hay bales disappear from the fields, school shoes must be bought, as must the 57th protractor set. I set about forcing my wild creatures back into their uniformed selves. Their souls don't quite fit, but order must return.

"I really don't want to go back to school …"

"No one does."

I don't look up from sewing name tapes. I don't take much heed.

"There are some really horrible rumours going around school about me."

"About what?"

"Nothing. I don't know. I really don't want to go to school."

Here, at least, I am on tried and tested ground. You haven't wanted to go to school since you were four. Ten years later, and you still don't want to go back to school. Transitional issues, night to day, home to school, holidays to term time. There was always a reason, and this time it happens to be about a rumour. I know what I have to do, I just have to get you over the threshold. You've never had a problem learning, you're a smart child – it's the inner workings of your peer group that you find unsolvable and while that may never be brilliant, bearable will have to do. Bearable means at least you are getting an education, and an education can springboard you into the rest of your life, where pecking orders and popularity matter less and it will be your turn to shine. Those whose school days are the best days of their lives are going to discover that in the greater scheme of things, school days don't last that long. It will be over soon enough and then you can choose your own path, your own people. We just have to get you to the end of the beginning, so that you can really start living.

The Sunday afternoon countdown is a precarious thing. We distract you all with the ultimate weapon: cake. We are driving through the town when you get the call in the car.

"Hello? … What?"

Something about the call distresses you. You go quite pink in the face, then the call ends.

"Who was that?" I ask.

"Someone asked me if this was the number of the local prostitute."

"What? A friend? A joke?" You say you didn't recognize the voice. "Take down the number. Let me call it back."

"No, no. Don't do that, it doesn't matter."

"It does matter. Why would someone do that?"

"I told you, there are rumours going around about me at school."

"What rumours?"

"I don't know." Creeping hostility.

"Is it because you went to the party?"

"I don't know."

It is hard to write tone – but take my word for it, this is said with undisguised loathing. I make the mistake of assuming that loathing is directed at me. I make that mistake a lot.

I berate myself for being stupid; I shouldn't have let you go. I suspected it was a mistake, but I also wanted you to go to a bloody party, for once, and simply be the girl who gets to go to the party. But it had been a risk, and it sounds like the risk had not paid off. You return to school, and whatever it is that is making you cross does not blow over. We live in the thick of your bad mood.

So much for no harm done.

NONCE

I try to tell you what I have done. We are sitting underneath a tree in an adventure playground. Everyone else goes off to play, but I stay back with you. This is my chance. I tell you that I have had an idea for a book. It is a book that explores the everyday issues of being a teenage girl while also examining mother–daughter relationships. I emphasize the problem of guys asking for nudes, repeating it over and over again and saying it is a main theme in the book.

"Girls who send nudes are stupid."

I am trapped. You aren't going to help me.

We were always told not to send inappropriate photographs, warned of the dangers, told of people whose lives had been ruined because of it. I am not denying any of that. What we were never told is what to do after it has happened. I've already done it and I know I have fucked up. I know that I have ruined my digital footprint. I don't need to watch another ICT video. I need some-body to listen to me, not judge me, and help me. So, I know that your generation don't really understand the concept of nudes, but you guys clearly got up to just as much inappropriate stuff. But I guess it scares you because it is unknown. Perhaps you don't even know what I mean when I talk about nude photos – because, to be honest, they aren't even nude. Guys send dick pics, so do girls just send photos of their vaginas? I can't speak for others, but I never did. Although perhaps I should've, because at least then nobody would have been able to identify me.

*

I get a Snapchat from a boy in my year. I had a crush on him when I was 10 and pretty much haven't spoken to him since. As soon as his name appears on my screen, my jaw clenches – I just know.

He has sent me four photos of myself, photos that he shouldn't have. Aiden has sent them to Liz. If she has them, then anyone could've seen them by now, and if they haven't seen them yet, then they are going to see them very soon. He won't tell me who sent them to him – he thinks it's funny. He is laughing at me. This isn't funny. I can't breathe. He doesn't know the whole story. Nobody is going to listen to me. This isn't me. This is me.

*

We are sitting in a cafe on the first day back at school and I am once again telling you that I cannot go back to school because there are these awful rumours going around about me, but I can't tell you what they are. I am hidden in baggy clothes that hang off me, but I am not prepared. You don't listen. You tell me that this happens every year and it is just back-to-school-nerves. I get in the car to be driven to school and my phone rings – an unknown number.

"Is this the correct number for the local prostitute?"

I hang up.

CAN I HAVE A WORD?

I continue life in the centre of your cross hairs. You scowl at me from behind the magnified teenage lens. Everything I do is infuriating and everything I ask you to do is resisted. I remember my mother losing it over wet towels left in puddles on the carpet. I stare at the wet towels on your floor and silently apologize to my mother. I can rationalize the towels, most of the time, but it is the rudeness I can't handle. There was no way my sisters or I would talk to my mother in that tone of voice. It's derisive with a touch of spite and frankly, it is stretching my patience to the max.

"What is the matter?"

"Nothing."

Then please, give us all a break and stop being so foul. Or if you can't stop, then go to your room and let us breathe less contaminated air. I wish I had the guts to say that. Instead, I tiptoe and pander and try not to set you off. The younger two need some lightness, to be able to chatter inanely about their day without feeling self-conscious or having snide comments thrown their way. They are an effervescent pair, close in age and spirit, loud, joyous, energetic … You wince at their high-pitched voices.

I take you to a friend's exhibition, but you lean against the wall, watchful, resentful and bristling with awkward nerves. On the anniversary of the Thursday we heard about my cousin's death, you and I decide to cheer ourselves up and go and see the musical *The Rocky Horror Picture Show*. The outing isn't easy, but at least I think I know why. Of course, I have no idea why.

"Roxy, please, what is going on?"

"Everyone is being horrible to me."

"Even the girls who came to your birthday?"

"Especially the girls who came to my birthday."

"Why?" I ask.

Silence. The music starts playing. You never answer.

Your behaviour is becoming exceedingly wearying and even the smallest thing feels difficult. We seem to be making more exceptions and more excuses for your mood, but regardless of whatever allowances are made, the mood continues to darken. It is draining and difficult and when we try to find out why, we are given nothing to go on. Frankly, I am not surprised people aren't being very nice – you are foul to be with.

I am at an afternoon concert that your school have put together to raise money. You are part of the group of singers. But while everyone is laughing and chatting – it feels like everyone knows everyone – you refuse to say hello to me. You won't even make eye contact. As I stand there on my own, I choose to pretend that I haven't noticed, but in truth, I am embarrassed, hurt and cross. Why do I bother? Why am I giving up an afternoon to support you when you don't even have the manners to say hello? It's just so rude. Have I mentioned that I hate the rudeness?

You sing beautifully. I always like to hear you sing, but you look so uncomfortable standing there that it makes it painful to watch. I wish I hadn't come and I escape as soon as I can. I am practically running when I approach the car. I can feel the adrenaline surge – and then your teacher calls after me. My head dips. I want to get away from here, away from this feeling.

"Can I have a word?"

DID YOU HEAR SHE …

Day by day I know the photos are spreading. I never see it happening, but I can feel it happening. Girls back away. Boys ask blatant belittling questions. Some boast they know who has them. I need to stop this. It is ruining my life.

It is 9 p.m. on a Tuesday. My knees are wet from the damp grass underneath them and his hands press heavily down on my shoulders. It feels very strange for my head to be at the same height as his waist. I try to move away, but he holds me down harder with his left hand and uses his right to clumsily undo the button and zip on his jeans. I don't want to do this. I tell him that I don't want to do this and I squirm underneath the weight of his huge hands. Why am I here? Did I really believe that he had just wanted to apologize? I had wanted to know how many people he had sent the photographs to. Instead, I am on my knees in the dark.

"Come on, Roxy, I know that you want to," Dan says. I protest and try to push his hands away. He laughs and grips my shoulder harder, pushing himself closer to me. I'm crying now, I feel weak and numb. I just shake my head. He keeps telling me that I want to.

I don't remember how I get away but I do remember running. I don't tell anyone about what happened, I haven't made it stop, I have made it worse.

I wake up on the worst day of my life and I cannot make eye contact with you. You roll your eyes at my rudeness, but it doesn't bother me. I know that there is no coming back from the hatred you will soon feel towards me. My housemistress calls me into her office as soon as I get to school.

"We know what you have been sending these older boys, Roxy. We are going to be investigating it more today and we are going through some boys' phones."

I knew that this was coming. For the past two weeks, I have watched while more and more people found out what I've done. I have seen the photos circulated to almost everybody. My friends have backed off. Every day, I have told myself that today will be the day that I tell you. I have needed you so badly.

"Girls who send nudes are stupid."

The words echo in my head. Now I am here. This is the moment that seemed so impossible for months. Everybody knows and soon so will you.

She recommends that I just go to lessons as normal and I will be brought in if they want more information. I nod my head and walk to History. I sit at my desk and while my teacher is rambling on about Cuba in the Cold War, I start to cry. It is not the cute kind of crying where I dab my eyes with my sleeve and sniff occasionally. Uncontrollable tears start to roll down my face and I gasp for air. Snot starts to spill from my nose. The teacher continues talking. I try to make eye contact with people sitting around me, begging them to help. They look away. Nobody says anything. I eventually announce that I am going to see the school nurse and the teacher visibly sighs with relief. I go to the nurse and collapse on her floor. In a 10-minute whirlwind, I tell her everything I have done. To a stranger, I utter the words that I have not been brave enough to say out loud to anyone up until this moment. She hands me a glass of water, but I am shaking too much to hold it. She puts her hand on my shoulder and tells me that she has to go tell the deputy head. A man. The rest of the day is insane. I am pulled into an office where they tell me what is going on.

"We are going through the phones and the photos. Luckily for you, we are not going to be contacting the police."

I sit there silently, trying my best to absorb what these men are saying. I should tell them that the boys at school did this to me. I should tell them that this isn't my fault and that I was scared. I should tell them that I am still scared and that these photos are everywhere. I should point out that I was 13 and they are 17, maybe 18, I don't know because I don't know them. I should stand up for myself, but I don't. I sit there as parts of me start to fade away. I am not strong any more, I am not smart any more. I begin to feel like the attention-seeking slut with self-esteem issues that these men are making me out to be. I pray that somebody will come to my rescue, but nobody does. I don't have the energy to fight this by myself; I am out of fight. I decide to take the insults, the punishments, the humiliation. There is little point in trying to tell people the truth. Nobody will listen to me, especially when the fantasy stories being spread by the boys are so much more entertaining. Apparently this random girl sent them photos without them asking, that's their story and they are sticking to it. To be honest, it is easier to be the school slut than to try to explain all the many complications that I am made of.

I have been sent to cross-country. I go up to the starting line in my trackies and they tell me that I have to strip down to these tiny running shorts and a see-through white top. I run past the entire school as they whisper and point. After the race, I try to catch up with the girls who used to be my friends, but they make up a pathetic excuse to not go to lunch with me. The deputy head tells me that he is going to tell you this evening. I walk into my PSHE lesson and everybody looks at me and goes deadly silent. I sit down at my desk and turn to face the whiteboard. Roaring laughter explodes from my mouth. I can't stop – I howl. "HOW TO USE SOCIAL MEDIA AND WHY SENDING NUDES CAN BE DANGEROUS" is the title of the PowerPoint for today's lesson. Everybody stares at the crazy slutty girl who has lost her mind, but I don't care. I haven't laughed in a long time, and this is so amazingly funny.

After classes end for the day, I am told that I have to stay to participate in a small concert because it is a charity event and I must contribute. You have come to see me, but I can't make eye contact with you. I don't want to stand up and sing. I want to run up to you and curl up on your lap. I want you to stroke my hair and tell me that my life is not over. I want to make the most of the last few moments before you find out. Instead, I just don't look at you. I can't look at you because if I do, I think I will burst into tears in front of all these people.

SEX, LIKES AND VIDEOTAPES

I don't want to go back in and I don't want to see you and I certainly don't want to play the proud parent at that moment, so I try to put her off.

"Can this wait, I've—"

"Shall we go into my office?"

Hmm. You are a pretty model student as far as academics are concerned, so I am not initially worried, but her evasive response trips a minor alarm. We walk into her office and she shuts the door. There are two other members of staff cramped into the small room. They are introduced to me in turn. The deputy head, also head of pastoral care, who I have never met, the deputy head of pastoral care, who I know by sight, and your head of house, who I know pretty well. It is quite an intimidating line-up.

"Please, take a seat."

This is not looking good. Me against three. The deputy head, the only male in the room, starts talking.

"It has come to our attention that Roxy has been sending photos of herself to boys in the sixth form," he says.

I note the plural. Boys.

I note that you have been doing the sending.

And I note photos. Again, plural.

You have been sending photos to boys.

You.

Have.

Been.

Sending.

Photos.

To.

Boys.

My first response is simply to buy time while my brain starts working. It appears to have temporarily shut down. I want to say "What?", but I don't want to hear him repeat what he said. I plant my feet on the floor. I breathe, I breathe, I breathe. While I do not understand the desire to take a photo of myself and send it, I am fully aware that a great number of people communicate this way. Boys and girls, men and women, are pinging their private parts all over the web. I am frequently told this is flirting in the post tech-rev age and I shouldn't over-react, so I try not to overreact. My adrenal gland is, however, overreacting. Breathe.

"Don't they all send pictures of their body parts? I don't understand it, but I know they do it."

He gives me a strange look, a mix of obsequiousness and pity. I don't like it.

"These are not parts."

You wouldn't be that stupid, would you? I don't say this out loud. But I have to say something.

"How do you know it's her?"

There is that look again.

"The photos are identifiable," he explains. Full-body shots. I feel sick. I've taken three hits in quick succession; I am reeling and in shock but trying really hard to think, think, THINK!

"How did you find out?"

There is some awkward shuffling about some story that it had only come to their attention because some of the female sixth-formers had heard things and were concerned.

"What things?"

"Rumours."

My heart sinks. *Mummy, there are some really horrible rumours going about me at school. People are saying horrid things about me. People are being really mean. My friends aren't talking to me …*

"So we investigated and we found the photos."

"Where is she?"

"Yes, it's a pity she's not here," says the deputy head, the only person who has been talking. The two other members of staff, the women, just look at me – kindly, forlornly, pityingly, with a pained smile, a gentle grimace. Internally, I am free-falling.

"She wanted us to tell you because she was worried you would be angry."

"I said I would go and get her," says the head of house, but doesn't move.

I'm not angry so much as confused, perplexed, upset, stunned – but you're right, it all balls up into a tight knot of something that feels remarkably like anger. I mean, in what fucking universe do you think it is a good idea to send anyone a picture of yourself and believe that it won't come back and bite you in the perfect Instagram arse? What had you been thinking? Why would you do such a fucking stupid thing? They are watching me. Think, think, think.

"We think it might be a good idea if she saw a therapist."

"A therapist?"

"Why does she feel the need to send such photos? We think it's evidence of some troubling self-esteem issues …"

"Yes, clearly, but wait, look –" finally the cogs are turning – slowly, but turning "– I think this has more to do with her peer group, I mean it's never been easy."

The deputy head seems perplexed.

"What issues with her peer group?"

Really? Where do I start? I look to your housemistress for backup and get nothing. So I plough on. Alone. From this moment on, I find myself alone often. Where I expect support, I find a firing line. Words tumble out of me, as I attempt to form a case for your defence.

"She's had her games kit cut up by the girls in her form, her uniform hidden, her perfume emptied over her toothbrush, her mouthwash used and spat back into the bottle, her phone taken and messages sent to a boy as if from her. We've been to the headmaster about it. During the summer holidays, she was disinvited to a party last minute, they abandoned her in a car park, she was devastated, she's had a really tough time breaking through the friendship groups. One boy slapped her around the face on a school trip –"

At last, something other than a benign, patronizing glaze registers on the deputy head's young face.

"Was that reported?"

It is the only time I see him looking genuinely concerned. I know then whose side he is on, and it isn't mine.

"She told the teacher in charge. Look," I say, wanting to get back to explaining my fast-forming theory, needing them to understand, "if this sixth-form boy, and I suspect I know who it is but I can't remember his name –" *mother-fucking bad-boy, the one with the looks and the reputation*, "– was showing her interest, then it would have been a coup she couldn't resist. That gets her in with the group, I really mean it, I think this has more to do with being accepted into the group."

They stare back at me blankly and say nothing. Do these teachers have the faintest clue about what actually goes on at school? I understand that in the game of social snakes and ladders, Dan is a long ladder. He is a dick too, but only through the parental gaze. I am trying to be open to your culpability – I don't much admire the parents who believe their child incapable of any wrongdoing. *Not my boy, girls will be girls, it was just a joke…* There isn't a crappy trope I haven't heard over the years to minimize the impact of one child bullying another and for the parent of the terrorized child, it is crucifying every time. So yes, Roxy should have known better and I will deal with that, but for the love of God, we are not talking about pupils on a level playing field. I am trying to give them context. The bad-boy sixth-former had a draw that would have been hard to resist. He has the power. I am so close to the edge of the sofa I might fall off. I am leaning in about to launch into my theory again, but I stop. They had said "boys" … was it maths geek Ryan as well?

"Who are the boys?"

"Sorry, we can't tell you that."

"Hang on, these boys have naked photos of my daughter on their phones but you can't tell me their names?"

"Data protection," he says.

The school protects them from the beginning.

I glance at the clock. I have to collect the other two – I don't know what to do. After a brief conversation between the teachers, it is decided that you should stay because there is some school event happening, I can't remember what, but they want you to get back to normal as soon as possible so it can all blow over as quickly as possible. As if that was ever possible. I walk away from the building feeling heavier with every step and I climb into my car. I'm not sure I've had enough time to build up the reserves in my resilience tank since the last blow a year ago. Foolish girl, foolish girl, foolish, foolish, foolish girl.

VICTORIA'S SECRET

I wait at my desk, I wait and wait and claw at my fingernails and chew on my lips. They said that they would come get me when the meeting is over so that I can talk to you. You have been in that room for ages and I cannot wait any more. I venture out and see that your car has gone. You've left. You've left me. You couldn't even look at me. You couldn't even take me home.

"Sorry, Roxy, we forgot to tell you that your mum has already gone. We think that it is important to stay to watch the charity football game and support your friends."

My friends. My friends who won't be associated with me. You left me.

I walk through the cafeteria to get dinner. At the moment, the girls in my year are going through a phase of wearing trackies everywhere to make the boys think that they don't care what they look like. I have found somebody with a spare pair so that I can blend in. I wear no make-up, my hair in a tight bun, I even walk around the outside of the hall rather than through the middle so that fewer people see me. I go up to the water fountain.

"Roxy, you are wearing your trackies so low on your hips, it's kinda slutty."

The girl who says this to me over my shoulder used to be my friend. I feel myself go cold. I want to disappear but we are being funnelled out to the sports field for the charity football match.

The charity is Young Minds. There is a rowdy crowd already there, six-foot men shouting and cheering. I see the large silhouette of Aiden. I see Dan dribble the ball to raucous cheers. The whistle blows on the sixth-formers' match. They are everywhere, clapping backs, congratulating themselves. They've won. I want to rear up like a frightened animal, dig my feet into the mud, snort and buck, but there is no escape. The teachers lead us forward to line the pitch. I am the cow. This is the abattoir.

Then I am standing in front of you in our dark cold kitchen. It is 10 p.m. and I am exhausted. I mumble through some of what has happened. I cannot say my whole story out loud. In fact, it takes years before I can say those words without them burning my lips. The last thing I need right now is to be questioned. I understand that for you this is the beginning of this drama, but it has been months of hell for me. You want to treat me like a stupid teenager, to tell me I fucked up but that I can talk to you. I am so far beyond that.

I was a stupid teenager, but I haven't been for months. I am now a bruised girl who has been thrown around and not listened to.

I don't need your help now, there is nothing you can do. I don't need my phone to be taken away and a lecture on my digital footprint. You don't want another drama and your eyes tell me that. You want to be rational and not dramatic. That is fine, I'm too tired to be dramatic anyway.

I feel numb.

Everybody wants to put me into a box so that they can bullet-point the reasons why I am in this mess. They want to list off my personality traits and put a label on me. Nobody fits into a perfect box, everybody has a complex personality and different reasons for why they get into similar situations.

At this point, it is easier to wear the label and sit in my box.

You are almost irrelevant at this point. It isn't my job to help you process this. You weren't there to help me. I trust that you will read parenting forums and online explanations and come up with your own reasons and your own box.

I know that you are angry and I am too tired to fight that.

I hand you my phone. Confiscating it is what you feel you ought to do as a responsible mother.

You accuse me of deleting the social media apps in order to hide things from you.

I deleted those apps a week ago when I started getting unpleasant texts from strangers calling me a slut.

Goodnight, Mummy, I am the stupid slut with self-esteem issues.

*

The next morning you tell me that I don't have to go to school if I don't want to. Despite the little blip in History class yesterday, I am still trying to be strong. When they see weakness, they start to rip away at you like a carcass. I really try all morning. I don't cry and I don't hide. At about 11 a.m., a boy in the year above tells me that the teachers are calling loads of people to question. It seems like any boy I have ever spoken to is being questioned. A girl then tells me that Liz is telling everybody what story to tell the teachers and she has power, so they are doing it. The story is that some random girl, idiot me, sent photos to Aiden, out of the blue, without him asking. In one carefully constructed lie, they are all absolved. I also sent them to loads of other guys at school. Liz has nothing to do with it. The school seems to not care at all about trying to limit the rumours spread about me; they are literally calling in all the boys in the years above me and telling them what I have done. I run up to Horseradish.

"Please, please tell the truth!" I beg him.

"Chill out," he says.

I don't know when they started dating, but he is pretty in love with Liz at this point. I can't do this any more. Everybody is lying and laughing and lying and laughing. I call you and ask you to come get me. You take me home. You take a phone call and I sit on the sofa with our dog and eat a whole ball of mozzarella. I can't stop crying. I have promised Ruby that I'll take her down to London for our cousin's birthday this weekend. I really don't want to go. On the train, Ruby asks why I don't have my phone, and I tell her it is broken. My dad is in London and he doesn't know what I've done yet. You want to wait and tell him when he gets home. I smile through dinner with him, knowing that tomorrow our relationship will change forever. I know that this is the last time he will see me as his little girl. I want to apologize and cry and explain, but I just stay as quiet as possible. I'm scared that if I open my mouth, it will all come exploding out.

I go shopping with my sister, my cousin, and Alex, who insists that we go into Victoria's Secret. She doesn't seem to think that the photos getting out is a very big deal. I think she's relieved that she has gotten away with it. She thinks I am overreacting. For her, there was no coercion, no threats, they were just having fun. I go into the shop and I can't breathe, everything starts to spin. The huge photos of models wearing practically nothing loom over me. I run outside and slide down the wall until I am a ball on the floor next to this homeless man. He tells me it is going to be okay. I can't cry because my sister is here.

*

I am standing on the platform waiting for the Tube, and when I hear the train coming, I step forward to the edge of the platform.

It isn't really a decision; it just feels so right. I stand so close to the edge that I practically feel the train brush past my cheek. It is the easy way out. I wouldn't have to face what I've done. It doesn't feel like I can go back to my life – it doesn't really feel like I am welcome there any more. It doesn't feel like this is going to all blow over and then I can go back to being me. Me. What even is "me"? I am the photos, I am the boys, I am all the names they are throwing at me, I am the picture that the school has painted and wrapped in a bow. I am a messy, attention-seeking, dumb teenage girl with low self-esteem. I am the girl that parents thank God isn't their child. Other teenagers can say at least they are not me. I am the train wreck that went from model student to stupid slut. I don't think I have the guts to actually end it, but maybe I do have the guts to keep going. Either way, I push on through.

I get home and sit at the outside table with you and Dad facing me. I have said to myself for months that I would rather die than have this conversation, yet here I am. Dad barely looks me in the eye throughout the whole conversation, but then at the end, he looks straight into my soul and asks, "Weren't you embarrassed? I would be way too embarrassed to send naked photographs of myself to anyone." Then we all hug and go and watch *Strictly Come Dancing* results. I feel surprisingly safe and normal; you both know and I am still alive, breathing. I thought that this would end my life, but I am still here and I feel like with you both on my side, there is a chance that I can fight this. You don't hate me, so maybe I am not as disgusting as I feel. This evening lures me into a false sense of security that comes crashing down as soon as I go back to school.

Part 4

MOVING ON …

I am sitting facing two of the same three teachers from that first hideous meeting, but this time I am armed. Firstly, I have names and I am prepared to use them. Secondly, my husband is sitting next to me. Is it my imagination or does everyone act a bit more respectfully when he is in the room? I look directly into the head of pastoral's odd man-child eyes and ask him.

"Between the two sixth-formers and our daughter, who do you think had the power?"

"We are not at liberty to discuss the boys …"

"They shared images between themselves and threatened Roxy if she didn't send more."

"For now, we are mostly concerned with Roxy's well-being …"

"Roxy's well-being has been shattered by two sixth-form boys. She was 13 when they asked for those photos."

"The most important aspect of things now is that we help Roxy to move on –"

"How can we move on if we don't acknowledge what happened?"

I can feel myself shaking, not with nerves, with rage.

"The boy who blackmailed her, Aiden, is a cousin of Liz, the girl who disinvited Roxy from her party and, as a result, left her stranded in a car park. Liz shared the photos and is now telling the boys what to say. What is the school doing about that?"

"Given the inevitable chatter, we are investigating as thoroughly as we are able."

Inevitable chatter is killing our girl.

"Roxy has been stupid," I say again, "no doubt, but the boys have been manipulative and the girl downright vicious. What is the school going to do about that?"

113

"We are not at liberty to discuss that …"

"We are concerned with Roxy's well-being …"

"Moving on …"

Moving on. It became their mantra. What a load of crap. I can see myself now, perched primly on the sofa, knees touching, hands folded, playing it safe. I did not want to rock the boat. I was trying to keep the school on side; I needed their help. Above all, I must appear absolutely and completely rational and in control of my emotions – because falling to my knees, pulling at my hair and wailing accusations that they weren't listening to me or acknowledging that my child had suffered a terrible wrong in a place legally required to protect her would simply get me dismissed as an irrational, overemotional, overprotective helicopter mother. That kiss of death and I would lose the power to affect change.

Your dad takes over while I visibly fizz with fury.

"Roxy told us that her maths teacher had seen the photos, can you explain that," he asks.

"Procedure," says the deputy head, "when looking at…" he is trying to find a palatable word. There isn't one. "There have to be two members of staff in these situations."

"Ok, but did that have to be her teacher, did they both have to be male?"

"He didn't look at them, he was just in the room."

We're not convinced but at this stage we feel it is the least of our many concerns. And then comes the kicker.

"Roxy will be issued sanctions because she has broken school rules about ICT use."

What?

"She is gated and we will get her to do some reflective work."

I don't even know what that means.

"This will have the added benefit of removing her from some thoughtless behaviour from some of the boys in school and serve to take the wind out of the sails of those boys who may be claiming they have been treated unfairly."

I find that hard to write now. Treated unfairly? Those *boys*. Were they even boys at that stage? Weren't they on the cusp of being adult men? Seventeen- and eighteen-year-old young men who played Top Trumps with naked images of my 13-year-old child feel like *they* have been treated unfairly? Why am I not dialling for a lawyer? Screaming blue murder? Throwing a stapler at the man-child's head? I wish I had. I am so sorry that I didn't fight harder for you then.

"I know she's been stupid," I say on repeat, "but she hasn't been cruel." Unlike Liz who spread the photos Aiden sent her. What I should have said was that malicious distribution of sexual images is a crime. Distribution of explicit images of underaged children is a crime. Instead I just keep saying Roxy's been stupid, but they've been cruel. They've been so much worse than cruel. The Deputy Head keeps ignoring me. Instead, he recommends a counsellor.

"… so *she* can explore why *she* feels *she* has to behave like this, so *she* can learn strategies for coping and changing it."

From that miserable week in September, it was all on you.

I have written this to you without the benefit of hindsight, but I would like to say this here. To the best of my knowledge, the boys weren't asked to change their ways. No one was asking the boy who coerced you to explore why *he* felt *he* had to behave like that, so *he* could learn strategies to respect girls of any age but particularly girls as young as 13. No one was asking the boy who blackmailed you to explore why *he* felt *he* had to behave like that, so *he* could learn strategies to respect girls of any age but particularly girls as young as 13. To this day, I have no idea if they were punished or if their parents were ever informed. Two years later, the headmaster said to me he wished he had expelled them both – and maybe he does, but he didn't. And anyway, two years after that, he retracted the claim that he regretted keeping them at school, so perhaps it just depends on who he is talking to. One of the boys was his rugby star, too good to lose with one more season to go, I suppose. Whatever the reason, the headmaster's regret came too late for us. It is only thanks to our 24-hours-a-day, 7-days-a-week vigilance and the choice you made to rebuild your life, on your terms, that his mistake did not end your life. It did, however, end the life that you knew. By failing to make an example of the boys' actions, he condoned it. I believe that while the school's fundamental mishandling of the situation didn't result in your death, it killed you in a myriad of other ways.

But anyway, moving on …

*

Two days later, I am in a Brazilian bar in West London with the mother of your oldest friend. The following day, my husband and I are due to fly to Ibiza for a weekend away with a very old group of friends. It's taken a year to plan. We are on our second margarita when I feel brave enough to cautiously, tentatively, bring up the subject of sexting and what has happened to you as a result. Both our daughters have been sending images in response to requests, and if the roles were reversed, I would want to be told. So, I tell. I was braced for indignant denial. Instead, she howls with laughter. At first, I am rather shocked. They – mother and daughter – laugh about it, she tells me. They laugh about the ridiculous requests her daughter frequently receives and how she fobs them off with zoomed-in photos of elbow creases instead of cleavage, knees instead of boobs, a lovely pair of blue tits …

The thing is, I don't believe that is all her daughter is sending, but it feels good to laugh. Perhaps I am getting too intense, perhaps it really isn't that bad. She thinks it is mad I am even considering not going away for the weekend. Her sister, a lawyer, joins us mid-evening and we both laugh as my friend re-enacts her group of mum mates mimicking the teenagers' sexy poses to show them how ridiculous they look. Her sister, ever the lawyer, goes home and researches the legal ramifications of procuring and distributing sexually explicit images of children. In the morning, she rings my friend.

We are on our way to the airport when my friend rings me.

"I've been rethinking our conversation. Sexting isn't funny."

"No."

"It is illegal to send, receive or store naked images of children. It is considered child pornography. You can get a record. Future employers check up on this sort of thing."

"Right."

I feel even more sick, if such a thing is possible. Like I've drunk far too much strong coffee and it is swirling around my stomach which is simultaneously in an octopus grip of panic. *Luckily for you we won't have to call the Police.*

"This is no laughing matter," she says.

We arrive at the airport. I look at your dad. Police records? Child pornography? Are we mad to go? We discuss it again.

On one basic level, there is the undeniable fact that you knew you were playing a dangerous game and did it anyway. You are simply too smart not to have known that and I am cross with that part of you. We had no desire to punish you for it, but we had no desire to be punished either.

"She's on DofE, with some nice girls," he reminds me. "So slap on a smile –"

"And fake it till we make it."

I finish the sentence for him. We've been giving you this advice for years. Turns out, it is much harder than it sounds. We get on the plane and pour alcohol into the hollow and although I smile, happiness is hard to find.

ORIGINAL SIN

I am now ill. All the pretending to be strong has actually made me sick. I can't not go to school because that would look like I am hiding, so I go to lesson with snot streaming down my face. On Wednesday morning, you and Dad go on holiday. Suddenly, there is no escape from the rumours and looks and whispers because I am boarding for a week. You just leave. You fly off on a private jet to a really fancy holiday that you have been invited on. I really don't want you to go. I can grit my teeth and get through the school day but now I am here 24/7. People are so mean. I walk past buildings and boys shout out the window at me.

"Go on, Rox, can I be next on the list!"

"Come on, Roxy, just send me something nice …"

"Why don't you just show us a little something now?"

From the girls, I get the usual bitchiness. The not-so-quiet whispers, the slut-shaming glares. These people don't even know me. When I walk into my study, everyone goes quiet, and these are supposed to be my friends. The photos spread through the whole school; most of the boys have them. Thanks to group chats, they reach huge numbers very quickly. The teachers tell me not to worry because they have deleted them off Dan and Aiden's phones. They are so stupid. It has been three weeks since we came back to school – everybody has them. I cannot describe how difficult it is to walk with my head high when I know the majority of the people I walk past have seen me naked. I am called into the headmaster's office on Wednesday to receive my punishments. They tell me that I am house-gated, which means that I can't leave the house apart from to go to lessons. I have to write a "self-evaluation essay", which consists of 10 questions that I have to answer, including:

- Explain why sending photos is wrong
- Why is it so dangerous?
- How would you handle this episode differently if you had the chance to go back?

I find out later that another girl in my year had been made to write one of these essays. Her "crime" was saying "fuck" on Instagram, once. As if our situations are similar in any way. So I am sitting in my room alone "evaluating myself". It turns out that this task isn't particularly good for my self-esteem, mood, emotions, or anything regarding my mental state. It is also clear that it hasn't been well thought through at all; for a school that prides itself on its pastoral care, my well-being doesn't seem to be particularly high up on their list of priorities. They seem to think that their main job is to stop me from ever sending photos again.

This is the first time I hurt myself. It is a pretty pathetic attempt at self-harm. Scraping away at myself with a blunt compass.

I have to go on my Duke of Edinburgh expedition with the whole year group. I am punishing myself. I don't let myself eat and I keep using the compass. I make myself throw up. I feel so weak that I struggle to walk, and my legs feel like jelly. I am annoying the others in my group, but I don't even notice them. I take every opportunity to cause myself pain. On the bus ride home, people fire spit balls at me with straws. They throw rolled up notes with "SLAG" written on them. The girls who had stayed at my house during the summer howl with laughter as the boys come up with more and more inappropriate questions to shout at me. Eventually, a teacher takes me to sit with the other teachers. I am numb to the pain that these people are trying to inflict. It isn't making me sad – I just feel nothing. The abuse from them has nothing on what I am doing to myself. I haven't slept in days, so I rest my head against the cold window and fall into a deep sleep.

By the time you get back from your holiday, I am a different person. You have missed the chance to help me keep it together. I have unravelled too much for you to swoop back in. I am a shell of your daughter and I don't want to be here any more. I am completely alone. Nobody at school will speak to me and you don't understand.

My final punishment is that I have to see the school counsellor about the "self-esteem issues" that I have.

CHILD'S PLAY

I am sitting in a warm, soft beige room facing a beige woman. I don't yet know if she is soft or warm. I am feeling unaccountably uncomfortable. Through a round window, I glimpse the sea and wish I could open the window and breathe less cloying air. This is the counsellor you have seen twice. Not for punishment, but because you have always been uncomfortable in your skin and I think you need someone to talk to, since you are no longer talking to me. What softening there was after our last hug has gone. It has been replaced by a brittle hardness. Crackling static. Acute child–parent hatred. When I ask you about school, you spit with shards of venom and withering looks of disdain; no one is talking to you and everyone is being mean and I should stop asking stupid questions.

The thin woman draws on a flip chart. It is a set of circles to represent a mobile hanging over a child's crib. She explains in the sing-song gentleness of a nursery school teacher (or psychopath) that every family operates in a symbiotic way – though she doesn't use that word, her vocabulary is more infantilizing than that.

"Behaviour of one," she says, "impacts the experience of others."

No shit. I don't say this out loud.

Instead, I attempt to give her a potted history.

My father drank heavily. Evenings were dictated by his mood. So when Roxy's behaviour became explosive around bedtime at the age of four, it was all too reminiscent of miserable times, and I dealt with it really badly. I personally did a lot of work unpicking why: I went to weekend workshops on intergenerational trauma and co-dependencies, read Al-Anon literature so that I was better equipped to understand why I had such a visceral reaction to walking on eggshells in my adult home. I even took a parenting course.

I know the clock is ticking. There is so much more to say, the issues at school, the bullying that I didn't know about, I need to compress 14 years of your life into the remaining minutes. It is impossible, of course. I can only hope she has the required academic rigour and training to understand.

"You are dealing with a 10-day-old situation," I conclude, "but trust me, we've been dealing with this for 10 pretty challenging years."

I sound as though I am exonerating myself.

"Roxy is whip-smart," I plough on. "Do not underestimate her. We need to help her get through this as unscathed as possible."

I want the counsellor to know you need help, not artillery, but I don't feel confident that she has heard me. I can see she is listening to me through a curtain of preconceived ideas, and it worries me. I drive away from the meeting with a real sense of disquiet, and – I don't say this with the artifice of hindsight – I knew immediately that when you walked into that room for counselling, I would be put on trial. The counsellor will be asking the questions, but the judge, jury and witness for the prosecution is a miserable, vulnerable, brilliant 14-year-old girl who is pleading for her life. I failed you by not listening to my gut instinct that day. No one knew you better than me and yet my intuition was telling me that in this arena, my testimony was deemed inadmissible. I should have asked around, I should have got a better recommendation. As far as due diligence was concerned, it was not nearly enough. I severely let you down. I'm sorry.

After the first appointment, you told me she was rubbish and you didn't want to go back. But you do because I think it is good for you to have someone to talk to. I am getting conflicting information from your friends and the school that you are making yourself sick, that you are self-harming. I pass on this information to the counsellor. I have seen no signs of either and the friends who are contacting me are the same ones you say are ignoring you, so the picture is hazy and I need someone to help us work out what the hell is going on. I do this because

I think it will help you limp through the final week of this miserable half-term. In a few days' time, we are off on holiday to a perfect place for you to regroup, reassess and recover. I am naively hopeful.

After the third appointment, however, things change.

"How was it?"

"Actually, she's amazing. I really, really like her." This is said in an inexplicably accusatory tone.

"Good, that's great," I say, staying neutral.

"She's really understanding and really helpful."

"I'm so glad."

"And she's really kind. She's a really good mother."

"Uh-huh …"

"She said I don't have to go away with you if I don't want to."

"Did she now?"

"I don't want to go."

I snap into a more alert state. Hang on! What? "You don't want to come to Zambia?"

"I don't have to if I don't want to."

That's not really accurate, we leave in two days, but I don't say anything. Instead, I ask, "Why don't you want to?"

Your tone slices like a razor blade. I think it is designed to.

"It's obvious we can't have a nice time together. It always ends in fights. We're not a normal family."

I bite my tongue very hard.

"I think I should stay at school."

"You say everyone is being horrible at school."

"I want to board."

"You're coming home."

"Why? You clearly hate it when I am home."

Things turn darker from this day forward.

NOW I SEE

I sink into the ugly floral chair that smells like old people and cheap perfume. There are inspirational quotes on the white walls that seem to be getting closer and closer. There is a smiling face on the clock that is shaped like the sun. The window on the door is covered in cardboard to block out the nosy eyes of my peers. The counsellor, Sally, sits opposite me in an equally ugly chair. Her face is round and her eyes are strangely out of proportion. Her lips are two thin lines tightly pursed together. She looks like she has just eaten a Tangfastic, but her eyes are trying to smile at me. Her neck is too long, she is too thin. She is wearing a gilet, skinny jeans and suede boots that come up to just below her knee. Her legs are crossed. I am slumped over like a typical teenager who is reluctant to open up and is being forced into counselling. When she starts to speak, it is clear that the deputy head has already told her what happened. Well, his version of what happened. Nobody knows what really happened. I try to order the words in my mouth into the truth, but I can't quite make it work. She dismisses my stuttering attempt to piece together my story. She doesn't want to hear it.

The second time I go, I try to look sullen and mysterious, I don't want to talk about the photos but I am grateful to finally have someone who is going to listen to me. Someone who might be on my side. She says she wants to go deeper, straight to the cause. Dig in to why I have these debilitating self-esteem issues. I'm not sure how I am meant to tackle that when I cannot even say what happened out loud, but I am still out of fight. I sit and listen to the jabbing questions that she throws at me. Intrusive, leading questions about my childhood. My parents. My sisters. My fears. With her questions, she begins to paint a picture of

124

blame. Without really listening to me, she tells me why I did what I did. Don't worry, she says, it isn't your fault. You are just a victim of your parents' decisions.

Wow. I breathe out a sigh of relief that I think I have been holding in for weeks. She is the first person not to dump all the heavy blame on my shoulders. She questions me more, mostly about my childhood. I try to explain that my childhood was privileged, good. I tell her that the messiness of my own brain was the only thing that made my childhood tricky. She nods and continues to question. Any bullying? I found the people at my school very difficult and people were mean, but I don't really understand if that counts as bullying. Her eyes flicker: a possible lead. Any traumatic experience? No. Did your parents ever hit you? I mean, yeah, but in a pretty standard way – I was a complete pain in the arse. Her face completely lights up. Bingo. She tells me that I was abused. She says no wonder I sent nudes with that kind of childhood. I can't quite see the link. I mean, there are a lot of things I can blame my parents for, but I don't think sending inappropriate photos is one of them.

The thing is, she isn't blaming me. She isn't implying that I am a slut, or a screw-up. I know that it is pathetic, but I love not having to take all the responsibility. After every session with Sally, I hate myself a little less and my parents a little more. She is my best friend. She makes me feel less disgusting. I take her hand and she leads me down the winding path of blame. I get lost. I get confused. She takes me back to when I was younger. My brain starts to run rings around me, taking me to places that I haven't been for years. I am so angry at you – how could you have done that to your poor little child? How could you have punished me for being so scared? As if my constant anxiety wasn't punishment enough. Then my brain goes one step further, and suddenly, I am scared of you. I am not a 14-year-old teenager any more; I am a toddler who you hit for being scared.

WHOSE LAND IS IT?

At the airport you are more jumpy than usual. You have the eyes of a sniper, scanning queuing masses, seeking out the enemy in the grass. You keep saying you don't want to go – you've said it so many times that I am inclined to agree. Once again, it is a reminder of your childish naivety that we'd get the money back (we wouldn't), that we could click our fingers and find someone to care for you, in this state, for 10 days (we couldn't). I trudge on through the airport. Just get you to Zambia, I think, and even one tiny spot on that enormous continent will work its magic. How can it not? There is wisdom in its soil, soul.

Why Zambia? Because years ago, I worked there and still have friends in the tourist business. We are staying in their house on the banks of the mighty Zambezi River. You do not want to hear how an elephant charged me once on the banks of Chobe River in Botswana, or that my friends and I accidentally swam where croc bait was left, or that on a trip to Tanzania our Land Rover rolled on the road into Ngorongoro Crater … you don't want to hear anything from me at all. In fact, I will go as far to say that you cannot enjoy this trip because it means so much to me. I had hoped the sound of the laughing hippos would reach deep inside you and pull you out of yourself. But they just scare you. Everything seems to scare you.

The trouble is, I don't believe your fear. I feel I am watching a well-orchestrated performance. Your anxiety has been weaponized and is aimed at me. I don't want to see the world through your eyes, so I turn away and you bury yourself in a miserable book about self-harm. I want to throw that book over the Victoria Falls.

"You should read it," you say. "You might learn something."

You should look up, look out, you might learn something. You will not ruin this; I won't let you. Foolish woman. I should have heeded my own words of warning.

For Ruby's 11th birthday, we are camping on a tiny island in the middle of the river. There is no electricity or running water. Elephants stomp through it at night. I love it. Ruby loves it. You and your dad are nervous. Reva is being stretched between two camps. I watch as you pull her in as an ally, but I can't quite work out why. You are rude, ungrateful, spoilt and appear determined to hate every second of whatever is being offered you, however wonderful – especially if it is wonderful. Maybe it's worse because it's Ruby's birthday and she is getting the attention and you don't like it. Bog-standard sibling rivalry, as old as the Bible, but it truly pisses me off. Are you honestly unable to see the bigger picture? I am close to breaking point. Scratch that. I am at breaking point.

"Put a fucking smile on your face, come down and join breakfast to open presents with your sister." I really do not care whether this will feel like sticking needles in your eyeballs, you will do it because it is the right thing to do, so help me God.

This is a tiny island, basically an elephant's stepping stone across a river. We sleep in the open under mosquito nets, so Ruby hears me forcing you to play happy families. She looks devastated; she already fears you don't like her and I have just cemented that fear.

I try to keep my eye on the vast horizon. Perhaps that is my greatest mistake. I should have taken an early bullet and fallen, perhaps then you wouldn't have had to bring in the big guns on the last day.

We are at my friend's luxury lodge having breakfast waiting for the transfer to the airport. The mood is tetchy.

"Be polite, remember the other people around you, *don't fight*."

We go to a raised deck overlooking the river and order breakfast. I can't remember why but Reva asks how her grandfather died. Your dad was only seventeen at the time. She is only nine, she doesn't realize that perhaps he doesn't want to talk about that and so I try to change the subject. Reva gets upset and it suddenly gets very tense.

You sit a few feet away, watching. Ruby vacates. She finds a swing seat on the floor above, but Reva follows her up.

"It's my turn, Ruby!" she whines. She is wheedling, moaning, raising her voice – literally everything I have asked her not to do. You continue to watch to see what I will do. I go up.

"Reva, please leave Ruby alone," I say firmly, through gritted teeth.

She argues back. She always does. Her strength is admirable when I am strong enough for it, but I have been worn down by a 10-day targeted attack. I snap.

"You are ruining everyone else's breakfast. No one wants to hear you fighting."

Reva digs in. The peace has been shattered. The breakfast is a disaster. Now I just want to leave.

"We're going."

Ruby leaps off and heads for the exit.

"No!"

"Reva, we are going now."

"No!"

"Put on your shoes and come with me."

"I WANT A TURN!"

Reva refuses to move, refuses to put on her shoes, refuses to stop shouting. I am so cross that I pick up her flip-flops and throw them at her and then I leave.

And you pounce.

This is the proof you have been waiting for. I am an unfit mother. Reva yells from the floor above that she has a bleeding nose. I walk away. I truly don't care. She has had about three a day. It's the heat. She's very good at dealing with the nosebleeds except when she is vying for a fight. I go looking for Ruby. On my return, I see you with your arm around a weeping Reva, her nose bloody, but nothing a wad of loo paper won't deal with. You look daggers at me. Nothing new. I am not even alarmed, just mildly curious as to where this newfound care for your baby sister has come from. It's been largely absent for nine years.

"You hit her with the flip-flop," you hiss. "What is wrong with you?"

"I didn't," I reply. I can honestly admit here that I wanted to. That's why I threw them down, that's why I left. I had reached boiling point and I knew it. I was so sad because I really love this part of the world, and I believed it would heal you and help us.

"You hit her and gave her a bleeding nose," you say, your arm still wrapped protectively around Reva, cursing me with your tone.

I really should know better than to argue back, it makes me sound childish and defensive, but I feel the need to defend myself.

"I didn't hit her."

"You hit her across the face with a flip-flop and gave her a bleeding nose," you say again, unflinching.

"I did not," I say again, fear quickly replacing fury. Did I? Did I hit her across the face with the flip-flops? Would I? Now I'm panicking.

I believe this is the moment we reach the point of no return. We are standing on the banks of the great Zambezi – if you listen, you can hear hippos honk, fish eagles dive, the waterfall roar – but it has proved to be no match for your hatred, which you have brought all the way from England. It has festered in the heat.

In Swahili, they say a lion's roar is a question and a reply. If you hear it, it makes sense.

Whose land is it? The lion roars.

Whose land is it? The lion repeats.

Mine.

Mine.

Mine.

I can see fiery flecks of hatred in your gold-green eyes.

"Well," you say, triumphant, "it wouldn't be the first time."

The lioness has landed her prey.

*

The journey back to the UK is horrendous. You shoot daggers at me every time I speak, so I retreat further into silence. I speak only when spoken to. The stopover in Johannesburg is interminable. I spend our last few dollars on a CD; I loathe airport tat, but it gives me an excuse to leave the table we are forced to huddle around. Proximity is painful. Reva is now your bitch, your fool – you are pulling the strings and she is dancing obediently. She has no idea what you're doing, but I do.

I keep going over the breakfast in my mind. Checking and rechecking my recall like an obsessive-compulsive person checks the gas ... how many times I revisited the same scene just to make sure I didn't, as you are claiming, hit Reva in the face with a flip-flop and give her a bleeding nose. I have to really ground myself, really concentrate, really think … I went upstairs. I was, I admit, furious – so is it possible that I did intend to hit her with the flip-flop? I cross-examine myself over and over. It is terrifying how flimsy my certainty is, I know I didn't do that, I know it, but I am not 100 per cent certain. I can see my raised hand, I can see the flip-flop bouncing on the sofa, I can feel the dam break and the sheer force of pent-up misery and fury burst out of me … so maybe, just maybe, it did hit her. I know I did not hit her around the face with the flip-flop as you are saying, but I cannot swear I meant no harm.

You are even more nervous as we take our seats on the plane for the last leg of the journey home. An overnight flight. You have the eyes of a sniper, scanning the passengers, seeking out the enemy in the grass. Your ears primed to the mechanical sounds of an aircraft readying to depart. Your head swivelling this way and that, craning to see out of the window. It looks exaggerated to me. Impossible not to notice. I choose not to notice.

"What if we crash?"

"We won't."

"But we could."

"We won't."

A lifetime of "What if?" questions. A lifetime of answering: Run the numbers. You're a smart girl, you're good at maths, run the numbers. But statistics don't matter in the face of fear. It doesn't matter that flying is the safest form of transport. It doesn't matter that you're more likely to win the lottery. The fact is *it could happen*. I'm not in the mood for the verbal dance.

"But what if we do?" you ask. Pale. Wide-eyed. Lip bleeding. Nails bitten to the quick.

"Well then," I retort meanly, "at least it will be quick." And the thing is, I mean it. It would be quick and it would be over. We'd be together. I am sorry to admit that the thought of eternal rest didn't sound so bad.

You look like I've slapped you.

Reva has another bleeding nose on the flight and I feel marginally vindicated. We go to the toilet together to mop her up.

"Reva, we need to go over what happened at breakfast."

"You hit me with a flip-flop."

"I didn't."

"You did."

"Reva, this is really important, we need to remember what actually happened. Did I hit you around the face with the flip-flop?"

She screws up her sweet nine-year-old face. "Hmm, I think you did. The flip-flop hit me in the face."

Okay, we are making progress. This is a question of intention.

"But I didn't hit you *around* the face with the flip-flop."

She sees the problem and, for the first time, seems unsure. Conversely, for the first time, I am sure. I think I understand.

"I was standing away from the sofa, my reach isn't that far. I don't think I could have."

"Maybe you threw them at me."

"Maybe. Sorry, Reva, I shouldn't have done that. I'm sorry I lost my temper."

She is sorry too. That's the thing about Reva: she erupts with no warning, but her fury dissipates with equal speed. I envy her that. My anger grows like cold mould into coarse resentment, which lays itself down like sedimentary rock in my soul. I wish I could blow ... No, I don't. That thought is terrifying.

We leave the cubicle relieved, having agreed that my intention was not to hit her or cause her a bleeding nose, that I threw the

132

flip-flops at her feet and that they may or may not have bounced up, but they probably didn't give her a bleeding nose. I weep with relief.

We sit, bleary-eyed, in a Costa Coffee at the arrivals gate. Early-morning stragglers float through a near-empty terminal. Your dad is leaving us at this point to go to London. I need him to make sure you know that the relentless attack on me stops here. He doesn't get cross with you very often; he is the maker of magic, the man who says yes, he likes treats and just wants his girls to be happy. I am the bad guy. There are few families I know where this is not the case. Someone has to be the disciplinarian. I doubt I have to list the chores, since the women reading this already know them, but it is the domestic detritus, the manners, the reading, the spelling, the teeth, the shoelaces, the nits, the thank-you notes, the tidying, the crumbs – on and on it goes, endless, every day, and our capacity to endure expands with every little job. Until it doesn't. On the morning of 26 October 2016, I had taken enough. I am done. It's not as if *I* sent the fucking photos.

The argument between you and your dad is neither subtle nor proactive. He is just cross. As cross and tired as I am. There is a little part of me that regrets asking him to do it, but there is also a part of me that wants him to know what it feels like because you turn your fury on him. This is new.

"Are you going to hit me as well?" you sneer at him.

"No," your father hisses back, "but you sure make me want to sometimes."

I know he says this because we can all hear it. He is incandescent that you have not acquiesced in any way. The shitshow continues. We stop for more coffee while we wait for our car and there, in yet another dismal Costa Coffee, I decide to confront you. Facing you, I say:

"I did not hit your sister in the face with her flip-flop, despite what you think you know, despite what she said, despite what you think you saw, it did not happen. That convenient tale ends now."

You really want to continue blaming me but you also want an out. I watch the conflict of interest flit across your narrowed eyes.

"Do you hear me? I did not hit Reva across the face with the flip-flop."

"Okay, okay …"

"Say it."

"You didn't hit Reva."

"Right. That's it. This ends here."

Maybe your dad's fury did work.

We make the 150-mile journey in silence except for one request from you. You want to stop at my parents' cottage and grab your bike, which is in their garage.

"It won't fit in the car. We have too much luggage."

"I really, really want my bike."

"It won't fit."

You glower at me again. You've never liked not getting your own way, but the bike won't fit and that is that. I am way beyond bending over backwards so that you get what you want.

THE SMOKE THAT THUNDERS

I am hiding in a book. It has become my secret place during this holiday. I can surround myself with stories of abuse, self-harm, rape and murder, and I feel less alone.

I am brought back to reality when you storm into the room.

"Roxy. Get out of bed. Come outside and put a fucking smile on your face. It is your sister's birthday. "

I want to smile and be happy. We are on this huge adventure, and I love adventures, but everything scares me so much. I don't see the fun and the excitement any more. I didn't want to come to Zambia because I knew I couldn't do this. I am too exhausted to "Fake it till you make it", which were your words of wisdom. I think that I am breaking.

I feel like I am starting to lose control of my brain. Like it is telling me what to do instead of the other way around. I think that my brain and I have always been in a battle for control, but now my brain seems to be winning. I am so scared and I am not sleeping.

I live in London but I live in the countryside. I am five years old but I am also 14. I am scared of you but I need you. I am a slut but I am also a victim.

"Mummy, I am so sad and scared. I feel these urges to cut myself, like I am being told to. I feel completely unsafe and I am scared. I think that there is something wrong."

Your eyes roll and your stare hardens and there is not an ounce of care in your body. You look bored. I should be over the whole photos thing by now. It doesn't matter that I was publicly humiliated, shamed, and disowned by all my friends. I am just being dramatic and you have no time for it.

"Stop being so selfish and come celebrate Ruby's birthday."

You are scaring me. Like you used to when I was younger, like Sally said. You are another thing to be scared of. I built up the courage to tell you how I am feeling and you have just shut me down entirely. I want to cry – but not in front of you. You would consider an outpouring of pain attention-seeking and weak.

"Roxy, be outside in five minutes. And take your bloody malaria tablet."

Then you leave. I ruin Ruby's birthday. Again.

*

A week later, we are sitting at the restaurant for the last meal of our holiday. Reva starts to have a tantrum and you are angry. I leave you upstairs with her and a minute later she comes down with a bleeding nose.

"Oh my God, what happened?"

"Mummy hit me with her flip-flop."

I ask you what happened and you say that you threw the flip-flop into her lap and it bounced up and hit her in the face.

My head starts to spin out of control. Everything Sally has been saying is right. You are dangerous – and because I didn't say anything, you have now hurt my sister.

The flight home is awful. I've never been scared of flying before but I am completely on edge. Every small bump sends adrenaline racing through my body. I think that I am going to die.

When we land at Heathrow, Dad pulls me over to one side.

"Roxy, stop being so awful and rude to your mum. God, I want to hit you so badly right now."

Alarm bells ring so loudly in my head that I feel dizzy with fear and panic. You are both dangerous. Sally is right. I am not safe.

TAKE FLIGHT

It is staggeringly beautiful autumnal weather. Trees glow, suffused with light and the sky is a crisp cerulean blue, so I make some calls and gather up two nice girls in your year to join us for tea in a cafe overlooking the marshes. The huge sky reminds me so much of Africa. This place has soul. The telling off from your dad and confrontation with me seems to have landed with you. There is a temporary reprieve in the hostilities – always helped by the presence of others. I am going to make sure we spend as little time as possible on our own until school goes back. It works. We actually manage to have a pleasant time. I debate with myself that perhaps all you needed to know was that you'd gone too far – and boy, had you gone too far.

The following day, with the weather still holding, I organize another outing. This time, we're heading to the beach to madly throw ourselves into the sea, then recover with a flask of tea and cake. We do this quite a lot.

"I don't want to go," you say.

"But we're meeting your friend there."

"I'm really sorry, I don't feel like swimming."

I hesitate. Something doesn't feel right.

"I promise you, I'll come next time."

It's your tone. It's sickly sweet. Immediately, I am dubious. Isn't it sad that I am suspicious of your friendliness?

"I don't feel very well either," says Reva.

I give in. If you stay behind, Reva can stay in bed. So Ruby and I head to the beach and then go into town to grab some food for dinner.

"Any requests?"

"Burgers," you say. Then, "Please."

I notice the "please". This is what I decide. You are making an effort to be pleasant. It isn't particularly authentic, and clearly you have to force the kindness into your voice and it's sticking in your throat a bit, but at least you are trying. All will be well. Perhaps Zambia worked its magic after all.

It's a 20-minute drive for a 40-second swim, but the hot tea after tastes divine. There is more science out there now as to why cold water reboots the system in the way it does, but all I know is that it makes me feel strong again, and I need to feel strong again. I had no idea how strong.

I know as soon as I walk back through the door that something isn't right. The house is too quiet. I go upstairs and find Reva still sitting in bed. She looks nervously back at me, her duvet pulled up to her chin.

"Roxy has gone for a bike ride."

"What? When?"

It seems you took off shortly after we left for the beach, leaving your youngest sister alone in the house for close to two hours. I go to your bedroom and notice immediately that the sleeping bag lent to you for the Duke of Edinburgh Award is no longer on the floor. My heart constricts. I take a breath and tell myself to stay calm, but I know on a molecular level that you have not "gone for a bike ride". The missing sleeping bag tells me all I need to know. I call your number. You do not answer. The sky outside is turning leaden grey, and I have a real problem on my hands. Ruby and Reva look at me, wide-eyed.

"It's fine," I tell them, but they are smart and are not convinced.

The following texts tell you, better than I can recall, what it is like minute by minute on our end, as it dawns on me that you are now a high-risk individual.

28 October 2016

17.52 *Im fine*

Answer your phone. 17.53
Where are you. 17.54

17.58 *Everything is just too much, i am so unhappy*

17.59 *I need some time and daddy was scaring me i dont wanna c him*

Where are you 18.03

I am driving around looking for you 18.03

18.10 *U wont find me go home. Im fine*

It is dark. Pls don't cycle in the dark. I will come and get you 18.11

18.12 *I am not coming home*

I have to know where you are and that you are safe. 18.16

18.16 *im safe go home*

I have to know where you are.

I wont come and get you but I have to know 18.17

18.19 *Idk where i am. But I found somewhere safe, im turning off my phone now*

I will call the police Roxy you can't stay out all night 18.20

Please please please don't do this 18.20

18.23 *Dont u dare call the police, they wont find me leave me alone i rly cant face everything. Anyway im just feeling sorry for myself aren't i?*

Find a signpost. Tell me where you are 18.23

18.24 *No go away, im going to sleep. I don't wanna go home*

I cant help you unless you let me 18.25

I am getting back in the car. Give me a sign post 18.25

18.26 *I said no. none of u get it, go away*

You are a missing child. I have no choice if you don't tell me where you are. There will be a search. 18.28

I am so scared just let me get you home. 18.29

I went and got you burgers. 18.29

18.29 *Ffs leave me alone. I am not seeing daddy he was scaring me. im staying here*

Daddy isn't here 18.30

Please Roxy. The girls think you've been run over 18.31

18.31 *But he will be tmrw. Everyone hates me im staying here*

No one hates you. we love you so so much. But I will start a search if you don't tell me where you are. Roxy I love you. I always have and I always will. 18.33

18.35 no go away ik daddy hates he said he wanted hit me in the airport. Just leave me alone tonight.

No in 5 minutes I have to call the police. Your daddy loves you more than anything in the whole world. 18.37

18.38 im not coming home tonight

Then I will take you somewhere else 18.38

18.39 im staying here

Are you at someone's house? 18.41

18.41 no everyone hates me

Who hates you? 18.42

18.42 im not replying any more,

Please just let me come and get you. we can deal with all of this together. We have love and brains and experience and friends. We can sort this. 18.43

18.44 no I just wanna leave

Rest in Peace, I think. Over and over. Rest in Peace. Not again. Not another. Not you. Please God, not you too.

Please roxy you are terrifying me. 18.45

LEMON SHERBET

I want to try to describe what it feels like to start losing touch with reality. I want to describe that feeling of not quite knowing what is real and what is not. I don't remember much. I have tried to make it up and describe my crazy in a literate way, but it doesn't work. I am not sitting in that field analyzing the voices in my head or wondering if the trees are actually speaking to me. It is just all very real. It is also so simple. This voice has told me that I have to run away, and then it is just a task that I have to complete. It isn't really crazy and chaotic and dramatic, it is just something I have to do. I do not bike away from the house at great speed, checking behind me every few seconds to see if I am being followed. I just bike. Then I just sit in a field. Then I just read my book and listen to music. That is my story of that night. I do not lie in my sleeping bag thinking about how crazy I am. I am not safe at home, so I leave. I know this isn't very exciting to read. I am tempted to fake some movie-like description, but I would be lying to you. I run away because I have to. There is no other option.

My brain has this control over me. I am an automaton just doing what I am supposed to do, but someone else is giving the instructions. It is scary, being a puppet, but my brain and I have always battled for control, so it isn't a completely new feeling. My brain is winning now. I was in danger, so I left. It is all very simple and straightforward and it makes so much sense. Nothing has been making sense for a while, but this does.

Sally has made it so crystal clear: bad childhood. Bad parents. Not safe at home. Must leave.

I guess what I am trying to say is that the things that look so obviously unhinged from the outside feel so clear. I have a plan, so I will complete it. It feels good to have a plan.

I packed a rucksack last night with a map, water, energy bar and lemon sherbets. I leave my nine-year-old sister by herself, grab my rucksack from the cupboard, take my dad's bike out of the shed and just start biking. I haven't really thought about where

141

I am going, I just need to get as far away as possible before you get back and realize I am gone. I bike in the opposite direction to school. At every crossroad, I take the turning that we take least often. I am excited and proud of myself. I have felt for so long that I am in danger and now I am escaping. I am leaving a place that I cannot be in any more. You hate me for the photos. I see how disgusting you think I am. I feel the hatred that you have felt towards me for so many years. Dad is going to come home and he is going to hurt me and you will hurt me and they will hurt me.

Eventually, I don't know where I am any more. When I think that you have probably gotten home, I find somewhere to hide. I go through a gap in the bush that lines the road. I am in a huge field. The land slopes down into a dark ditch with trees. This is okay. I can do this. It gets dark early. I lay out my sleeping bag and curl up inside. You text me, but I know that no matter how nice you are to me on text, if I go home you will be so angry. Both you and Dad are so angry at me.

999

Dialling 999 is the most extraordinary thing. It is something so familiar, embedded in the vernacular, but to do it, to actually dial those three numbers, is shocking, I couldn't believe I was doing it: 9. 9. Hover ... really, really, my daughter has run away and I am calling the police, for real ... 9. I am patched through, and with my larynx dry and twisted deep in my throat, I try and explain the situation. All I want to do is cry, but that is not going to help them or you, so I swallow the feelings down, and tell the operator that I don't know where my child is. Outside the kitchen window, there is nothing. There is no light pollution here. Out in that blanket of darkness is my child, the same child who was too scared to stay in bed in her own room, in her own house … all I can see is my own reflection clutching a phone and speaking impossible words. In the next room, two little girls in fluffy dressing gowns watch *Daddy Day Care*. I can't protect them from this. I am so sorry this is all happening to them when they're so young and last year was so difficult, and now I have to ask them both to be more grown up than they should have to be.

I call your oldest friend, Alex. I bring her up to speed as quickly as I can. Immediately, she offers to try and get you on the phone. I wait, feeling sick, for her to call me back.

I wait, but I can't wait, I can't do nothing. I call the counsellor and ask her to try.

I wait.

I call you.

I text you.

I wait.

Finally, my phone rings. It's Alex.

"She's in a field, in a sleeping bag under a tree. She doesn't know where she is."

This beggars belief. My child, so afraid of sleep, so afraid of danger while asleep, is in a field? In the dark? It is so unbelievably dark out here. The absence of light feels eternal.

"She says you had a fight," Alex mentions.

"We didn't have a fight," I correct her. "We'd been playing the guitar and singing before going to the beach. She was in trouble before, but not today."

There is a pause.

"She told me that it wasn't normal, what our mothers did to us."

"What we did?" My mind is racing to fill in the blanks.

"She said you slapped her and gave her a bleeding nose."

"When she was eight!"

Alex has known me her whole life. We have spent a lot of time in the bowels of each other's families, and I don't think she would condemn me as a violent mother.

"Somehow she made it sound like that happened tonight. Like that was why she ran away."

I am now more confused than ever. "What the fuck is going on, Alex?"

"She says she's not coming home. Are you sure there wasn't a fight?"

"There wasn't a fight." I see lights outside. "I've got to go. The police are here."

The police are here. Holy shit, the police are here. Immediately, I tell them you've answered the phone. They look relieved.

It is utterly surreal introducing the two uniformed men to my two pyjama-clad children. The girls are so sweet, they are so worried, they are being so brave. I send them back to watch more telly as I bring the officers up to speed. It makes me feel sick, retelling this tawdry tale. Young girl sends photos to older boy, boy trades photos, blackmail follows. That is basically what happened. The very first question the policeman asks me is …

"Did the school report it to the police?"

My thoughts start racing again. *Um, God, not this, please don't condemn her. Child pornography. A police record.*

"I didn't think it was a police matter, she was just –" I've got to get a grip, think of something to say. PC Dawson must have seen the fear flash across my face because he instantly, and gently, puts me right.

"She's not in trouble."

Inhale. Exhale. I want to cry. I mustn't cry.

"It is illegal to send explicit images of a child, regardless of who sends it. However, children are very, very rarely prosecuted because, usually – and it sounds likely in this case – they are the victims, not the perpetrators."

I blink at him.

"It wasn't her fault," he says. "She needs to know that."

I go over what he has said in my head. *They are the victims, not the perpetrators. It wasn't her fault.* What the hell is wrong with me! Of course it wasn't her fault, of course she needed to know that ...

"We are dealing with rising weekly cases of this nature," he says, glancing around our lived-in kitchen and seeing the situation with his well-trained eyes. "A young girl or boy falls into the trap of sending an image of themselves naked. This is a child pornographic image and it's illegal. Immediately, that image is used as leverage to gain more images. Threats of exposure are always part of it, which makes it coercive. The threats continue until the images are distributed, discovered, and their life as they knew it is over."

Sounds horribly familiar. And then he says something I will never forget and probably why I continue wading through the painful molasses of writing this book.

"The reason why it is so important we are informed," says PC Dawson, "is not to help the child who has been exposed – sadly, it is too late for them, as the images are already out there. The reason we need the schools to tell the police is to protect the next child from falling prey to the same behaviour because we know that unless stopped, there *will* be a next child and the crimes *will* get more severe."

I think I stop making tea at that point and just stare at him.

"So what happens? Are they arrested?"

"Very, very rarely. We prefer to visit the perpetrators and explain to them in no uncertain terms that what they are doing is distributing illegal images of children and, as a result, face being placed on the sex offenders' register. That usually works."

So simple. So effective. So obvious. Why hadn't that happened?

"We need them to know what devastation they are causing – and they are. Last week, we responded to a call exactly like this one."

Except that girl wasn't answering her phone, she wasn't in a sleeping bag in the dark under a tree – she had hanged herself in the neighbouring barn. She was 15. The officers tell me this story because I am still partially apologizing for wasting their time. It is this wonderful, kind, effective officer who finally impresses on me how very serious this situation is. Children die when photos they have taken of themselves fall into the wrong hands. They die because they took the photos. Self-blame and crucifying shame kill them, but the shamed should be the people who coerced them into taking the photos in the first place and the ones who shared them without permission.

I watch the officers go outside, taking their full-beam flash-lights with them, and head to the barn and outbuildings.

I watch the beams of light illuminate the waxy leaves of the giant laurel outside the back door. My mind sees you hanging from every branch. Shame kills.

The police come back in. Ruby finds a recent photo. I give them your mobile number. I do these things as if they are normal, but they aren't normal. I've just seen actors do it on TV, and I try to emulate the characters I most admire. I will not be the wailing banshee – I won't do that to my other two daughters – but I feel like I am cracking up, a term I now fully understand. The crack starts in the rib cage and sounds, to my mind, exactly like a crab claw being split open. I have cracked. Rip my heart out.

The police leave after telling me they may send up a search helicopter. I text this information to you because I know you won't want them to do that. What if someone died because a helicopter wasn't available to them because they were out looking for you? I hope this will shake you. After the police leave, I send another message to the counsellor. I threw her Saturday night into disarray when I called her and asked for help. By this time, I believe you know the police know because they have texted you and you know about the helicopter, so perhaps you feel you have no choice. As long as you are communicating with someone, we know you are alive. Your dad arrives after a hideous journey from London, receiving miserable updates from me with no good news. He walks in the door.

"Anything?"

I check my phone. Nothing. So just before 9.30 p.m., I text the counsellor.

Anything?

Talking to her…. Shes safe x

I immediately wonder why I had to ask for that information rather than her telling me, but I meekly type back a thank you. I look at your dad, sorry that he's had to leave final audition decisions for the new show he is producing only to arrive back as the drama ends. Maybe I overreacted. Maybe I should not have called the police. The self-doubts and mental doubling back begin instantaneously.

Then the counsellor texts:

I'm going to pick her up x 21.38

omg amazing will tell the police now 21.39

147

Yes – don't let the police go after her or it may spook her. I'll update you later x

Got it. 21.40

I am so obedient. Then we wait, with only conjecture and second-guessing to keep us company. The girls are happy to see their dad, but we are preoccupied and I have no doubt we fail to comfort them. All we can do is tell them she's been found and is going to be picked up and is fine. What we don't tell them is that a woman we barely know is driving around in the dark, trying to locate a child in the dark, and is then going to take her home. It was a long hour, adrenaline pumping through the system but nowhere for it to go except round and round in booming pulses through the solar plexus.

Hi Gay. We are home and Roxy is fine. She is staying tonight and I'll give you a call in the morning. 22.30

I update the police and they say they will go and check on you. PC Dawson explains that sadly in some cases the people who "rescue" runaways are in fact the ones pulling the strings. The darker side of life is illuminated. They call back and confirm you are safe. Your dad and I look at each other. It is midnight. Seven hours of hell followed by another seven hours of sleeplessness.

It is four in the morning. Your dad and I sit with our backs to the Aga, whiskies in hand, trying to work out what the fuck is going on.

EMMYLOU

I can't go home. Dad is coming back tomorrow and I am not safe. He said he wants to hit me. I can't go home. Sally is right. For somebody who has always been scared to sleep by herself in the dark, I can't believe I am here. With the light gone, the field seems bigger. The ditch about 300 metres away feels like a black hole. I read my book. Every time I hear a car drive past, I turn off my torch and hold my breath. I don't want to be found. I am not safe. Your texts scream at me through my phone. Everything is always screaming. I put my headphones in and turn on my old iPod Shuffle. I listen to the Emmylou Harris album *All I Intended to Be*. I used to listen to this album on repeat when I couldn't sleep. Emmylou feels like a friend.

You call me. Alex calls me. Sally calls me. Alex calls me a lot until I finally pick up. She might understand. Her mum used to hit her, maybe she will understand that we are not safe. I tell her hurriedly that what they did to us, it isn't okay. They were not supposed to do that. Sally says that we are not safe. Alex is confused, she doesn't agree with me, she doesn't know what to say. She mumbles for a bit and then I realize that she is probably spying on me for you. She is not going to help me – she wants them to find me. I hang up. The field is trying to trick me, but I know that it isn't real. It keeps making things look like something else. You tell me that the police will send a helicopter. No. No. No. This is the place where I am safe. I do not need to be rescued.

Sally keeps calling. I don't want to speak to her. She told me to do this, she told me I am not safe. I am protecting myself and my sisters. When she rings for the twenty-first time, I pick up. She tells me that she ran away when she was 14. She says that now I am even less safe. She shares with me that when she ran away, she was sexually assaulted by nine boys at the same time. I don't understand, I am so confused. She told me that I wasn't safe at home and now she is telling me that I'm not safe here and I need to go home. I don't know what to do. I don't want to be raped by nine boys and I don't want to be hit by my parents. I desperately look at my map to try to work out where I am, but everything feels so jumbled and I can't remember which turnings I took. I try to focus on the road names, but Sally is so loud on the phone and the noises from the bushes are so loud and the wind is so loud. I do my very best to explain where I am. I don't want to go home, so she says I can go stay at her house.

As soon as she hangs up the phone, I am terrified. The noises which I had blocked out now make me shake and breathe very fast. Every time I hear a car approaching, I pray it is her. I am not safe in this field with the black-hole ditch. She arrives. My dad's bike doesn't fit in her car, so I leave it hidden in a bush. Her house is warm and cozy. Her son is there. He is only a little older than me. He looks at me like I have just escaped from a psych ward or I am a rare and dangerous species. I don't care. Six months ago, I would've been so embarrassed that a teenage boy was seeing me in a tracksuit with no make-up on and twigs in my hair. I am too exhausted to be embarrassed. Two police officers come to see me. I am so embarrassed that I cannot look them in the eye; they know what I did. They ask me why I ran away. I say that I don't know. I tell them that it was just a mix of everything. I feel Sally staring at the back of my head, but I don't even mention you.

The police officers tell me that the school should have reported what the boys did. They tell me that it wasn't my fault. They tell me that the school lied: I would not have been in trouble. They tell me that I am the victim. I do not know what any of this means and I don't find it helpful. I am so, so tired. I just want to go to sleep, but when I get into bed my mind starts racing. The dark is playing its old tricks, making me see shadows that aren't there. I read the book *Scars* for the third time. I trace my pathetic cuts with my finger. I don't want these superficial lines any more – I want to slice through my skin with a blade. I want to feel the sting before blood starts to seep out. I want to watch as the blood just keeps oozing. I want the cut to be deep enough that the blood flows out of me. I want to pick at the scabs in the morning, making it bleed again. I drift off to sleep tracing the purple, bloody road map that I will create.

RABBIT HOLE

With gritty eyes and a hollow tremor that I learn to live with for a long time, I text the counsellor. It's early, but your dad and I don't dare take a step without consulting her. She tells us that you are still asleep and that you want some time apart from the family.

"It doesn't make sense," I say from the beginning. "School is where all the horrible stuff is taking place – all the name-calling, being ignored by friends. It doesn't add up."

"Something has happened to Roxy. I am close to finding out what."

"Okay, okay, whatever she wants." I feel sick just thinking about what that might be. I put your sisters in the car and we decide to go and walk the dog through the stunning woods near school. I choose this wood very specifically. Anywhere else, we risk bumping into people, but the school is deserted on a Sunday. You are holed up in a village on the coast, so the coastal path is out of the question. I am trying to remain undercover, which is difficult in a small community.

There is one other car parked near the entrance to the wood, overlooking empty sports pitches. One. In the back of it sits …

"It's Roxy!" cries out your youngest sister. My head whips round. You can't make this shit up. There you are – so small, so frightened, so not mine. Our eyes meet. I am not sure who is more terrified. I feel the compression of panic grip my chest. I want to fling open the door and pull you back from whatever miserable place you've gone to, I want to run. I don't know what to do. I try and slam the ancient Land Rover into reverse, but it's a beast to drive; I stall, I sob, I can't breathe, I tell the girls "It's okay, it's okay," I get the car started again, I reverse, the counsellor gets out of the car, my hand is trembling so much I can't get the window down.

"I didn't know you were here. We're going, we're leaving," I say. I can't do this …

She says something about her son doing tennis. He doesn't even go to the school, so what are the chances? What are the fucking chances?

"I didn't know, I didn't know …" I am sobbing now. Great chunks of undigested feelings convulse out of me. I've got to get a grip for the other two. I drive away.

"I'm okay, it's okay," I tell the girls. "Roxy's okay …"

It is so not okay.

"I'm sorry," I say, "I'm sorry, girls …"

"Roxy was crying," says Reva. We are all crying. What has happened to my family? This is fucking nuts.

Many months later, you tell me that the counsellor had suggested that I was somehow tracking you, that I had followed you to the car park. It didn't occur to me until writing this book what a deeply suspicious suggestion that is. She had made it clear you did not want to see us or be with us and we had to respect that or risk you running away again. So why would I then turn up unannounced? Secondly, how could I? You had an analogue phone, a brick, the "punishment" phone that could not be connected to the internet. I wish I had been able to track you. Then I would have come to find you under that tree; I would have put you, the sleeping bag and your dad's bike into the car and driven you home. Perhaps we would have avoided the shitshow that followed, because the shitshow that followed made what had happened up to now child's play.

In a bizarre way, it is child's play. You don't know this, or I hope you don't anyway, but you are now in control. You pull the lever that says jump, and we jump. Two steps forward, three steps back – we are moved like terrified pawns. "We'll do anything," we plead, "just let us have our daughter back." This takes many phone calls in which the counsellor tells us about what happened to her when she ran away, about the problems it caused with her parents when she returned, so getting this right is really important. We agree. We'll agree to anything.

A meeting is set up for later in the day so we can decide what will happen now. We are told that the counsellor is very close to uncovering the cause of your deep, deep unhappiness, she holds the key to why you want to disappear, the horrific thing that we know we don't know because we know the photos aren't enough to explain what is going on. We sit in the headmaster's office, bracing ourselves for the very worst. These are the things I am waiting to hear:

You've been raped.

You've been sexually assaulted by a person in authority.

You've been sexually assaulted by another student.

You have had consensual sex and are pregnant.

The counsellor leans forwards. I think my heart ceases to beat for a millisecond.

"Roxy told the police that she ran away because she is afraid of her father—"

I leap to my feet, shouting.

"THIS IS BULLSHIT."

Now, I am in no way my most rational self, I've barely slept, but this … Come on. I can't help it – I pace madly, speaking loudly, too loudly (I am now the hysterical mother I have tried so hard never to be; I should have let the banshee out earlier, the time for politeness is long over).

Your dad tries to pull me down. They all look a bit shocked. I really don't care.

"I've been waiting to be told our daughter has been raped!" Tears sting as the fear gets lodged in my throat.

"He would do anything for Roxy," I shriek, still too loudly, still pacing the room. It's true, sometimes it's even annoying – but hey, fathers and their first-born girls … I get it.

"He wasn't even there, this doesn't make sense …"

The counsellor continues. Clearly, I am irrational, prone to furious outbreaks, can't control my anger, probably shouldn't have reproduced, this is what I think they are thinking as I sit back down. The judgement rises like heat off a desert road. She silences me with one fact.

"Roxy has threatened to run away again if made to come home while her father is there."

Your dad and I look at each other. What kind of surreal performance is this? I know what this will do to my husband. He arrived in my life relatively empty-handed; we are his everything.

"Roxy has a problem with me," I insist. "Not her father and nothing that hasn't been going on for years. This doesn't make sense, him leaving is mad."

But your dad wants you home and if that means him leaving, then leave he will. I cannot believe what he is agreeing to. This is too terrible to witness. He hasn't done anything except tell you off for behaving like a foul, ungrateful, rude teenager. Hardly radical or original, it happens the world over. I have a nagging feeling we are missing a trick. I have a sickening feeling we are being played.

The counsellor tells me not to ask questions and give you space. She also tells me again that when she returned home having run away, her parents never asked her anything, which she interpreted as disinterest. When, years later, she asked them about it, they said they didn't think she would want to talk about it. She also told me she'd been sexually assaulted when she ran away. At the time, I didn't really care what she was telling me, it was only later that I wondered whether that was appropriate. I know now it isn't. It certainly made deciphering her advice harder.

"Just follow her lead," she advises.

Staggeringly bad advice. Your lead was leading us further down the rabbit hole.

It is dark and cold outside, and we are waiting for the sound of tyres on gravel that will announce your return. An invisible force is scooping out my insides like soft ice cream, starting with my solar plexus. Scoop, scoop, scoop. I try to refill the hollow with deep breaths of healing air, but the hollowing continues: scoop, scoop, scoop. The counsellor hands you over, you look to her for reassurance, she encourages you forward with comforting eyes that say, "It's safe". I look to her for reassurance too. Really? Has it come to this? It feels like we're trapped in a grotesque play. I half expect the counsellor to give me an exaggerated "she's behind you" panto wink, but she just smiles benignly. There is an awful awkward greeting in the hallway. I hold a rigid body in my arms for a moment, but it's clear you don't want to be held, certainly not by me. You seek out your youngest sister and brush past Ruby. So, the battle lines remain the same. Shame, because your greatest ally is sitting in a cold barn near my parents 45 minutes away in absolute pieces.

You look about, seemingly mystified, like you've never seen the inside of the house before. I am not taken in for one second.

"Where's Daddy?"

You sound oddly confused, as if you didn't know he wasn't going to be home on a Saturday night – but you know where he is because you have banished him there. I can feel anger seeping through my feet, creeping up the veins, polluting, toxic anger. If it gets to my heart, it will kill the love. I squash it back down with all my might, but I don't think I am mighty enough. This is going to be an agonizing evening. Sympathy is going to be hard to find, so I will fake it. I will fake my way through making supper, lighting the fire, watching *Strictly*. I will smile and speak gently and serve you whatever you need. But inside, hot fury is starting to bubble. I have to keep leaving the sitting room to go to the kitchen on some pretext, but actually I just need to breathe, to scream silently. I have to stop staring at you with utter incredulity and distrust. If your aim was to disarm me, you have succeeded. A song comes on: 'Love Potion Number 9'. It is a favourite of your dad's. You and he sing it a lot. I can hear you and your sisters singing along, what a sweet sound, what a sweet scene, and yet … I send a long text to your dad, but I can shorten it to three letters for you:

WTF???

These thoughts keep swimming around my skull: what madness is this? This is nuts, none of this makes sense, what IS going on? Of course, now I realize I had already answered my question. You do not make sense. You are nuts. You are mad. It's so obvious, looking back. I would put it a bit more delicately now, now that I understand what mental illness really looks like, but that night I knew nothing. Still, even in my ignorance I figured out delusion was the only answer that made sense. The trouble was I could not compute that it applied to you. So while I kept saying to myself, *This is nuts, this is mad, what madness is this?*, I did not think it. I did not accept it. In fact, I probably fought it, because that would make you mad and madness was a far more terrifying foe.

Reva has a party on Sunday, so I put you and Ruby, along with the dog, into the car. I tell you we are going for a walk. Which is true. I do not tell you we are going to my parents' house for that walk. You are livid when you figure it out, but I drive on. I need some time to think, I need to talk to your dad alone, I need to claw back some authority because I know, I *know*, that you are not afraid of your father, so something else is going on and we need to work out what that is – and fast. You tell me I am not allowed to take you places you don't want to go. You give me this list of your rights that I am somehow breaching, but as shaky as I feel, you are still the child and I am still the parent. Perhaps I am running to my parents because the truth is, I simply don't know what else to do. You want to call the counsellor. I tell you that isn't really appropriate on a Sunday.

I leave you with your grandparents while I go and check on your father.

"How the fuck have I ended up the bad guy?"

I wondered in that moment, and many since, how is it that I've been the bad guy for 10 years but as soon as it was his turn, he fell to his knees, shot through the heart. I grab his strong arms and pull him up.

Now is not the time. He needs to use that incredible brain of his and help me think. We need to think, or we might lose her.

We make a plan. You dad will not spend one more night away. He isn't guilty, he hasn't done anything wrong and allowing that narrative to gain weight is dangerous. I give you a choice. It is a choice I will insist you make.

I do it in the car on the way home. I am calm, clear, considered and contained. I grip the wheel. I am hanging on by a thread.

"Your dad is coming home tonight."

"Then I'm leaving."

"Fine. We would rather you stayed. But if you really feel you can't, then you can go to a friend's house or school."

"I'll go to a friend's house."

"Okay, but I will have to inform the mother."

"No."

"Then it is school or home."

"School."

I know I am pushing this hard and fast, but I don't want you pulling all the levers any more. I call the housemistress immediately and she says she is happy to have you.

"Why did you do that?" You are furious. "I hadn't decided. Not completely."

None of this is a surprise to me. I've taken a gamble and it pays off because, after going back and forth several times, you decide to stay. I knew you would, because school on a Sunday night is a bit grim and the food isn't great – but more than anything, it's because I know the accusation against your dad is false. You love your dad as much as he loves you, but perhaps you thought he could take it. More likely, you weren't thinking, you were just clawing for breath, the way a drowning person can pull their rescuer down into the depths with them.

Your dad comes home, we all sit down for supper, and he and I look at each other over your head and communicate silently. We've been through hell but are none the wiser. Still, you're home, the girls are safe and we can now put all of this behind us.

LOVE POTION NUMBER 9

The next morning, Sally says that we have to go to the supermarket. I ask to stay in the car so that I don't have to see anybody from school. She insists I come in. I am a floppy teddy bear being dragged around the supermarket by the wrist. She speaks to everybody and I stare at the floor. Maybe she wants people to see her with the broken girl that she is saving.

Then we go to the playing fields to drop off her son. The playing fields where I used to laugh and flirt, where I would kiss boys, where I had my first cigarette, where Dan touched me, where the whole school watched me run cross-country in practically nothing, the playing fields where I hid during lunch. As I stare out the window at the school I have to go back to tomorrow, your car pulls into the car park. You have been following me. I can't breathe. Sally betrayed me. I feel this magnetic pull towards you. I need to hug you and cry to you and tell you that I need help. I need you, but I keep my seatbelt on. I tried to ask for your help before, and you couldn't listen. You have come to punish me. She tells you to leave and, as we pull away, I see you put your face in your hands and start to cry.

Sally has gone to tell you and the school why I ran away. I don't know why I ran away, but I know that I am not safe. I watch *Pretty Little Liars*. We've never had Netflix, so this is exciting. Her son makes me a wrap for lunch with chicken and cheese. He is careful to not come too near in case he catches something. I don't think about how life will be when I leave this warm house. School starts tomorrow. I try to persuade myself that people will have moved on and that there will be a new drama; but I know that this isn't true. I will have to see the boys every day. I will be reminded that my friends aren't my friends any more. Walking alone, a thing that would've terrified me last year, is going to be my new normal. Home is scary and school is scary and my head is also scary. Sally says that she has the answers. I so need answers. The school tells me that I can board for two weeks.

I go home for the night and my dad goes to stay somewhere else. As soon as I step through our front door, I miss the warmth of Sally's house. Our house is dark and cold and it is where bad things happen. You are also cold and angry. Always so angry. You don't tell me where Dad is. I miss Netflix. The dog is allowed to sleep in my room. We watch *Strictly*, and a couple dances to mine and Dad's song. Music has always been our thing and I feel so proud that he thinks I have cool music taste. I feel blessed when he introduces me to his favourite albums and artists. I feel like a genius when I correctly identify which artist is singing a particular song; even prouder when I point out that it is a cover and who the original is by. Last summer, he gave me the *American Graffiti* soundtrack and told me he'd give me £20 if I correctly told him the best song on the track. I spent hours listening to each song and analyzing them with great detail. I devoured the lyrics and rated the songs. Eventually, after hours of thinking, I said to him, 'Love Potion Number 9' - and he opened his wallet. The happiness I felt is indescribable. Now, as we sit here, one of the couples spins around the dance floor to 'Love Potion Number 9'. It is a sign. It is going to be okay.

Looking back, I just wasn't really there. I remember small patches of what happened but I cannot explain any of it.

Part 5

WHO ARE YOU?

The phone rings. I put my coffee cup down and push myself out of the chair. I feel 104 years old, but all three girls are at school, your dad is back in London for work and it's a bright, blue-sky day.

"Hello, my name is Freya Lynn and I am a youth worker from social services."

I go cold all over.

"The police passed on the case ..."

She is speaking kindly, softly, but her words land like hammer blows.

"This is a routine follow-up ..." She wants me to know that the interview is informal but essential in a post-Rotherham and Rochdale grooming scandal world. The girls in South Yorkshire, Manchester and Birmingham who ran away from their abusers told the police at the time it was because they were in danger – being made to do things, being exploited, plied with drugs and alcohol. Instead of believing these "troublesome" girls, the police handed them straight back to the households they'd run from. The 2014 Jay Report concluded that an estimated 1,400 children in Rotherham alone had been sexually abused. So quite rightly, protocol changed.

The domestic situations of all runaways are now fully investigated.

I try to sound like a good mother as I fill in the blanks. It is starting to run off the tongue rather than stick in the throat as it used to.

"Roxy's reason for running away makes no sense. Her father wasn't even at home."

"This is routine," she reiterates. "Nothing to worry about."

I feel sick with worry. We are being investigated by social services. Holy shit, we are being investigated by social services. I call your dad and tell him the sorry news. We are being investigated by social services.

We are hurtling down country lanes during the first lunch break of your two weeks under the protection of the school because you want to go and find your dad's bike. We have been deemed the danger because of what you told the police, and yet I can still take you out at lunchtime on a fool's errand which will lead to nothing but more upset. Who am I to point out this anomaly? I am no longer in charge. My right to parent has been suspended while under investigation. I can't help thinking, as I grip the wheel and head off down another lane that looks exactly like the previous lane, that this is what you wanted all along: to board. It's a shit way to get what you want, and now you are stuck in a place where there is no escape from what has happened. How can that be a good thing? I look at you sideways as you scan the hedgerow for something recognizable. I don't know who you are any more. Even if we find the random bush, down the random lane, that you may or may not have biked down, the bike won't be there. It's an expensive bike and it will be long gone. While that is exceedingly annoying, it isn't as important as getting you back to school in time to see the counsellor at 2 p.m. She continues to assure us that she is very close to unveiling the root cause of your erratic behaviour, because it just can't be that you are afraid of your dad. It can't.

We fail to find the bike. We're late for the appointment. You want to know why I am so tight-lipped. Who are you to ask me such a question? I have no idea what to say to you any more, I have no idea what I am allowed to say to you any more. You don't let up. You push. You keep asking.

"Honestly, Roxy, I am mystified by what you told the police about being afraid of your father."

"I never said I was afraid of him."

"You did. That's why Daddy wasn't at home, that's why we are being investigated by social services."

"I didn't tell the police anything. I told them I was fine."

I watch you walk into the appointment at the health centre. I simultaneously check that you go where you say you are going, while wondering if you should be going in there at all. The adrenaline running through my system makes me feel sick all the time; my heart beats out a warning code, but I don't know what I am being warned about. The siren bellows, but for what – fire, flood, fatality? I am beginning to have my doubts about the counsellor that you now hail (her bill to rescue you came to £650). No doubt she earned the money, but I feel she has handed the controls of an armoured tank with a myopic field of vision to a 14-year-old girl who is scanning the horizon for a target, a reason, an excuse.

The school reports to us, telling us you are fine. Better than fine – you took part in the Halloween party and you appear more settled than before half-term. We are not fine. We are deeply unsettled. Then I get a text from maths geek Ryan which is so odd and disconcerting I forward it to the counsellor. Your dad tells me not to worry; he tells me it's a sideshow, but it freaks me out. More things don't stack up. If you've told no one, how does Ryan know, and why is he still texting me? And if everyone is ignoring you, why is your friend passing information to this boy in sixth form? And how can you be at a Halloween party, yet tell us you haven't left your room? Later, he texts again, begging me not to tell you he'd been in touch. He phones a couple of times. Your dad tells me not to answer.

On the day of your interview with the social worker, I have to go to London for work. It's a meeting that can't be moved. While I am away, you go and see your sisters. Ruby tells me you took Reva aside and told her a "secret" that she is not allowed to tell either of us. I talk to Reva. I know she worships you, and I can tell she is happy to be in your confidence. Reva won't tell me what you and she talked about because she says you will give her hell if she tells me. We discuss that, currently, things are too serious to be keeping secrets. Eventually, Reva tells me the secret is that you are seeing a social worker. I try to see the significance of this. Why the secrecy? Unless it is designed to divide and conquer, unless it's designed to pull Reva in … Reva, I see now, told me just enough to make me feel I had the answer, but I only had an answer, not *the* answer. The answer would have told me you were checking your facts, lining up your ducks, doubling down. Then Ryan leaves another message telling me that he was worried – you told him you just wanted to go and say goodbye to your sisters. I get more messages from him. Alarming ones about self-harm and being sick – and yet, the school insists you are doing much better.

I hurry back home.

On the weekend, you choose to go to see the musical *Chicago* with your dad. I take the other two to the fireworks. Somehow, it has become the fifth of November. People are smiling and making "ooh" and "aah" sounds and drinking mulled wine. I try and mimic them but I feel hollow on the inside. You and your dad have a nice time, he tells me later. You talked a bit about what was going on during the drive, but we had been repeatedly advised not to push, and he didn't. You two went out for a burger and backstage after the show. Almost normal, except for the Damoclean sword hanging over his head.

In the morning, what little charm was there has gone. You say you want to go to school early even though rehearsals for the school musical don't start until later. You need monitoring, so instead we all walk the dog. It is pretty painful, you with your earphones stuck in and wearing the wrong shoes, the wrong jacket, protesting with every silent step. So when it starts raining, you and your dad retreat to the cafe. Dad is no longer the bad guy, I note.

While you are at rehearsals, I go and visit Ryan at his home. I am now the one sneaking around behind your back, trying to piece this mess together. We sit in the smartly decorated sitting-room and he says the burden of knowing everything is getting too much – but when I press for details, he is obtuse. He says a girl has told him she thinks you are self-harming. I've seen no sign, but everything is so muddled and mixed-up I have no idea what is really going on. The kid clearly has a crush on you – perhaps he just wants to be involved, perhaps he feels guilty for asking for a photo back in the summer, perhaps he thinks you will kill yourself and he will have blood on his hands. I think now he is trying to make amends but doesn't quite know how. Later, he texts me to say that you have read his texts on my phone and now know I went to see him. You are furious about that.

We are both getting more suspicious of one another by the day. Nothing adds up. I can't work out what is going on, but it is making me very, very nervous. I change the passcode that I had put on my phone and tilt my phone away from your beady eyes when I open it. I add a passcode to my home computer too. Sad that it has come to this. When I try to talk to you, you tell me you don't have to answer any of my questions. There is a boulder between you and me. When I look at you, all I can see is the boulder. All I can see is everything that is getting in the way, getting in the way.

On Monday, the social worker calls. Unfortunately, she can't close the case.

"What? Why?"

In view of what you told her – we can't know due to confidentiality issues – a formal interview will now take place in our home.

Once again, my heart sinks through the floor. This is a feeling that is impossible to get used to.

"It doesn't make sense," I tell the social worker. "She and her dad went to the theatre. She chose to come home for the weekend. How can you still think she is at risk? I don't understand." I can hear pleading, needling, in my voice.

She explains as gently as possible.

"Everything Roxy said tallied with what I understood about the situation. However, at the end of the meeting, when the interview was effectively over, I did ask her if there was anything else she wanted to tell me. I did tell her at the beginning that whatever she told me I may have to take to my superiors."

I understand social workers are trained to fish with the greatest expertise and the gentlest of methods for a channel of communication with children who are suffering at the hands of the people who purport to love them, who are supposed to "look after them". It is not easy to get a child to tell on a parent or family member, especially if it is a parent or family member, so this last question, set up in the safest of spaces, is designed to draw out murky, toxic secrets that some children are forced to carry.

I am not allowed to see you but I go to school to meet you because you need to top up your phone. This is getting more unfathomable by the minute. We are civil but brittle when in the shop, but back in the car I can't hide how I feel.

"Why do social services still think you are at risk at home?"

"I told her that I wasn't frightened of Dad." You say this in an oddly friendly tone, like it was exciting news, almost like you had righted a wrong.

"But at the end of the conversation, when the social worker had said it wouldn't go anywhere, you told her something." I knew I shouldn't be asking, but I asked anyway. This dance was getting too macabre.

"She said it wouldn't go anywhere," you state emphatically. I look at you. You are a child and you don't understand. And the scary thing is, you think you do.

"What did you say?"

"All I said was that I wasn't worried for myself, but I was worried about what would happen to Reva."

I cannot believe what you are saying. Suddenly this is about Reva? I try to understand what you mean, but you just flare up, then you talk about how I slapped you in the face. Your new, shiny, staggeringly effective weapon switches to automatic; it is firing without prejudice, at random.

"My childhood was violent."

It is almost like you are tasting those words for the first time. Something is happening to you. I am watching it happen.

"There is something wrong with you. Something needed to be done to stop it," you continue.

"What are you talking about? Your childhood was not violent."

"You slapped me and gave me a bleeding nose." How easily this rolls off the tongue.

That happened once, when you were eight, and it in no way explains all of this – meaning the accusation against your father and the photos, but we are still not allowed to mention the photos.

You start firing another round.

"When your cousin died, all your attention was on that."

Really? I have to defend that?

"Well, yes … it was kind of important—"

"You did nothing about the boy who groped me in year 9."

Okay, so now, maybe, we are getting somewhere. I reach over to you, but you cry and tell me not to touch you and you leave.

I remain in the parked car. Breathe. Think. Breathe. Think. This is about me now? Or Reva? Or is it about the boy who groped you? I try to remember. The school did not inform me – you did, one evening, as we sat on the sofa. You told me he'd put his hand up your shirt. Did something else happen? Something worse? I wait. I suspect this isn't over yet.

Fifteen minutes later, you get back in the car. I try to offer you a way out of the maze you are building around yourself. I drop breadcrumbs.

Come on, Roxy, come back to me …

"You can tell me – whatever it is, however awful. What can we do to help you?"

But there is a shift now: cooler, colder. You say you're fine, that you're not depressed but that no one is talking to you (I don't entirely believe this) and that the name-calling is continuing (this I sadly do believe; boys are shits when they want to be, but hey, it's all banter, right?). I tentatively return to the topic of something happening after my cousin died, something you didn't want to tell me because I was so preoccupied. I apologize again for this, but my attempts backfire. You storm out of the car and this time, you don't come back. What madness is this? I keep asking myself that over and over. But it didn't matter what kind of madness it was. It was madness, and that should have been enough.

CUT, EAT, SLEEP, REPEAT

I go to school on Monday morning with a suitcase. I am boarding for two weeks so that social services can investigate you guys. I am so confused. I am sad to leave you but I know that I will be in danger if I stay. I also know that you are not dangerous, but that knowing is smaller than this terrifying feeling. Although I know that my parents are not abusive, I also know that I am going to be hurt. And Sally said that my parents are bad, so now it all makes sense. Being at school is awful, but I am scared of home. At lunchtime, you call me and say I have to help you find Dad's bike. It was a present. We go to the place where I had hidden it, but there is no bike. As soon as we pull up to the field where I had set up my sleeping bag just a few days before, I feel sick and comforted at the same time. This little place had felt so big and dark and complicated. Now, in the daylight, it is just a little gap in a bush. The field had felt endless and now it seems so small and simple. I can't believe that the bike is gone. You are so angry. Your face is scary. I so badly want you to hug me, but your eyes are so full of hatred. I want to cry but I wait until I am alone again.

I am now at school 24/7. There is no escape from the looks and the whispers and the shouting. I am always alone. Lessons go by in a blur, while I sit at my desk waiting for an opportunity to sneak to the bathroom. Halfway through *Strictly Come Dancing* results at home the other night, I had gone into the cupboard and taken one of your screwdrivers. I can now unscrew the blades from pencil sharpeners. The cuts are deeper and cleaner and the blood is a bright red. When I am walking around school and I feel scared, I put my hand into my pocket and hold the blade as tightly as possible. In lessons, when I cannot cut, I use the blade to shave away at my fingernails under the desk until eventually

I get to the skin underneath the nail. I cannot put that pain into words. It is excruciating.

I walk down to Reva's school and intercept her as she is walking to her lesson. I pull her to one side. I need to ask her if you actually hit her with a flip-flop. I am beginning to doubt myself: I am worried that I have chosen the wrong danger. I know I am in danger, but what if my parents aren't it? She tells me that everything she said was true. You hit her around the face with a flip-flop and gave her a bleeding nose. I tell her that I am sorry and I hug her. I stand outside Ruby's lesson and peer through the window. She sees me and waves, telling her friends that I am outside and have come to see her. I give her a hug and then I leave.

I don't go into the dining hall much because I can't face the looks, but when I do, I am sick straight after. I don't think I am fat or anything – it has nothing to do with hating my body. It gives me a sort of relief. In the brief seconds after I cut or I am sick, I can breathe. I don't blame my friends for bailing. I wouldn't want to be friends with me either.

The only person I speak to is Ryan. I wouldn't say speak exactly, he stays on the phone and we sit in silence. I think he feels guilty that he played a part in this. I don't know how to explain what is happening.

My life is very linear right now. Wake up, cut, eat, puke, cut, lessons, cut, lessons, cut, sleep. Well, sleep isn't coming very easily to me at the moment. The night-time is the worst. Even though there is nobody to tease me or jeer at me in this dark room, my mind tortures me. I distract myself by reading the same books again and again, but my brain is like a beast. I try to tame it, distract, it but it has this overwhelming force. It can take me anywhere and it loves to go to scary places. It is taking over. Even at night, I can feel the looks and the gossip. I feel like there are people watching me. I am scared again of being kidnapped or there being a fire. I plan my escape routes, but it brings less comfort than it used to. Most nights, I only get a few hours of sleep and they are interrupted by dreams and this feeling that there is somebody standing next to my bed watching me. I feel like as soon as I close my eyes, I am vulnerable, so I keep them open. Even when my whole body is desperate to fall asleep and I feel myself slipping into rest, I force myself to trace the letters of the book I am reading. Keep reading. I sneak to the bathroom, constantly looking around for scary faces in the dark corners. I splash my face with cold water and stare at my face in the mirror.

You are guilty, my reflection says. *You deserve this.*

I go back to my book. I do deserve this. I listen to Emmylou Harris some more.

THE SLAP

Your dad and I start to free-fall in panic. We are plotting a downward trend with every appointment you have with the counsellor Sally, and the ramifications with the social worker are deadly. You have two more sessions booked with her that week. It's like being faced with a runaway train.

This is part of the email he sends to the counsellor after another lengthy, panic-stricken discussion.

… Both Gay and I are worried that Roxy is getting herself into a dangerous corner. As the stakes get higher, she faces a choice of either backing down and revealing the hollow-ness of the accusations, or of battling on and increasing the stakes. Her counselling with you started in order to try and address the issues revealed by the photo texting in the summer. She has found a kind place of refuge and through that she has discovered a convenient target for her rage – her parents and her "violent" childhood. She regards your non-judgemental response to her narrative as a validation of it, and it is rapidly becoming the scapegoat for all of her troubles over the last year …

The words of a desperate father trying to stop that runaway train from disappearing over a precipice – or the plea of the guilty?

At 15.26, I get a text from you.

I am miserable.

I don't remember if I respond. You can't keep punching me and then asking me to pull you up.

The social worker arrives the following day, file in hand, and we sit at the kitchen table, pour coffee, swallow back bile. Our interview will take 90 minutes. I am grateful that we got the social worker that we did because she turned out to be heads and shoulders above anyone else. Who gets assigned to what case is random, but with Freya we got lucky. I know of two families who were not so fortunate and were dragged through hell by overzealous social workers who did much more damage than good. The head of the school that the younger two are at is fearful on my behalf because he has seen more cases like this go wrong than right. So I say again, we got really lucky because our social worker made a hugely positive difference to our troubled family of five.

During the meeting, we go through as best we can the time that has spanned your life: the sleep difficulties, the problems at school, peer-group issues. I tell her about throwing the flip-flops at Reva and the bleeding nose, then I take a deep breath and tell her about the night I slapped your face and gave you a bleeding nose six years before.

"I am pretty sure she was eight. We were staying at our old barn. It had big windows, was in the middle of a field, and was surrounded by inky black at night. She had come into my room several times and I would take her back to bed. Around four in the morning, she reached a new level of hysterical, and I made a decision to slap her around the face to shock her out of it. To make it stop. It was one purposeful slap across the cheek and it worked. It wasn't pleasant, I'm not proud, I wish there had been another way – but honestly, exhausted at four in the morning, I couldn't think of one."

The social worker watches me. I feel like a well-rehearsed fraud. I go on.

"Unfortunately, the slap caused a bleeding nose. I'm not sure if it was that or the slap that switched off the hysteria, but it did stop. We mopped up the blood together, I said sorry, and I was really sorry but she was calm. The shock of the slap calmed her down."

The meeting goes well over the 90 minutes, but even so, I am only offering her a sliver of the pie. I tell her your version of things are always coloured in the negative. Always have been and it was hard to always react generously when we were told how terrible things were. Working out the difference between perception and reality is difficult, so when someone like a therapist comes along and tells you perception is reality, well then hey presto, that makes you right, however skewed your thinking. You will think I tell the social worker this to cover my own poor parenting, but we are fighting for you because we need her to know that this situation is complex and if we take a wrong turn here, the damage will be long-term and far-reaching. I can't rule out fatal.

Then the interview takes an unexpected turn – and yet, it's not unexpected at all. While the social worker sympathizes, she wants to warn me that once her case is submitted, there may be a request to interview Reva. Why Reva?

"Roxy has implied that she is in danger." This is what I mean when I say you are shooting from the hip. Well, I won't let you take Reva.

"No." I know how guilty this makes me look, but I feel we have jumped through enough hoops. I will not jump through this one.

"You can have access to all school records, you can talk to my family, Reva's teachers, doctors, friends, anyone you need to in order to build up a picture of who my family is and how we work, but you will not speak to our nine-year-old child."

Sometimes you have to listen to your gut instincts. I wish I had listened to them more.

Freya, the social worker explains the catch-22. She informed you that, although the case was closed, whatever you added would have to be passed to her superiors and could involve the police and social services. This you appeared to acknowledge, and then continued to imply that you were worried for Reva's safety.

"If she had been so worried about her sister's safety, why did she leave her alone for two hours to run away?" It doesn't feel like a winning blow.

Meanwhile, another email from school comes in telling us how well you are doing. Well, bully for you – we are on our knees.

At 5 p.m., the social worker calls. She cuts to the chase. No further action will be taken. Reva has been taken off the at-risk list. They are completely satisfied that Reva is in no danger from us and as far as the Child Protection Team is concerned, the file is closed. However, she would like to come and see all three girls. She thinks she can help them all process what they have been through. I sink to my knees and thank the universe for sending me Freya Lynn. Of all the professionals we encounter, Freya is immediately reassuring and speaks to us like human beings being tossed in a storm. Her words flash in the darkness, a reassuring lighthouse that gives us fleeting moments of hope.

The family session with the counsellor Sally arrives, the make-or-break moment after which you decide whether you will return home to us, although of course you already have been home for the weekend in the middle which included a theatre trip to see *Chicago*. If it so pleases you, some rebuilding can then commence. We are under strict instructions not to ask questions or have any physical contact. I mean, man am I losing my patience with this head-tilting, sickly sweet, oversharing counsellor. She says she is here to help us heal our family, but I wonder if she isn't here to hurt. If priests can abuse boys, and family protection officers can abuse their wards, if neonatal nurses can kill babies, if aid workers can swap food for sex, then is it beyond the imagination that a family therapist can shred a family? It is not beyond mine.

Your dad is terrified. I am too, but not of her, of you. You have no idea how powerful you have become. Or do you?

We learn absolutely nothing except one perfect gem from the counsellor:

"The threat of violence is violent."

That is surely true when applied to domestic violence, coercive control, protection rackets, any number of hideous actions we commit against one another, but not to overtired parents who just wanted a fucking moment at the end of a long working day to sit down, uninterrupted, and pretend there was still some resemblance of a relationship between two once-happy-go-lucky people who are now utterly and entirely drained of life. You got in trouble because you didn't stay in bed and whatever you say now, you did not say then that you believed you were going to die in a fire, be kidnapped, be stolen, die or suffocate. All you said was that you couldn't sleep, night after miserable night. Well, that was certainly true if you were standing on the staircase. So, back to bed you were sent. Sometimes you were chased up the stairs, sometimes you were shouted at, but mostly you were taken back up and the reading, tickle, backrub routine continued until one of us went back downstairs and then, footfalls on the stairs, "I can't sleep." School was tricky for you. Home was tricky for you. It was tricky all round.

Of the many parcels of wisdom that were bestowed on us by the multitude of professionals we consulted during the previous 10 years, Professor Tanya Byron's explanation of safety held true. Whatever we did, she told us, we mustn't let you rule the household because, conversely, that would make any child feel less secure, not more. However tyrannically a child acts, they don't actually want to be in charge because then they wonder, "Who is looking after me?" But here, today, the counsellor has put you firmly in charge. We are not allowed to speak until spoken to. Trouble is, you're not really speaking, so frankly the whole thing is bollocks. The counsellor indicates that we should try and comfort you, so I end up sitting on the floor at your feet. The symbolism is not lost. You dominated the household for such a long time; I am loath to return to that dynamic because that would be feeding the beast and the beast is growing. When the session is over, in which we have learnt nothing, discovered nothing, progressed nowhere, you are signed off, and we all go home. Brilliant.

On Wednesday, 16 November you are sent to the nurse. You call me from there and tell me you don't know why you've been sent there. You sound very frightened, very young and very alone. I sit in my friend's house in London and listen to you breathe while dinner goes on in the other room. I cannot describe the abject loneliness this has thrown us into. It feels like no one understands, no one can help and it hurts. It really hurts. The following day, we get a call from school. They would like us to come and get you as they can no longer guarantee your safety. An email arrives from school with a helpful link:

mind.org.uk/information-support/types-of-mental-health-problems/self-harm.

"Any other advice?" I ask.

Don't leave her alone.

Right.

LONELY

I am reminded of how long nights are if you aren't sleeping. When I was younger, I used to find the 2 a.m. to 5 a.m. slot the hardest. That is when people who stay up late have gone to bed and people who wake up early are still asleep. Then the sun would start to come up and I could persuade myself that it was safe to get the much-needed two-hour sleep before I had to get up for school.

Now, I am still finding the 2 a.m. to 5 a.m. slot difficult. I feel the morning looming ahead. The morning comes with noise and punishment. The sun rises with a voice that questions if I will be able to get through another day. I get out of bed and wonder if today is going to be the day that breaks me for good. Then a sarcastic voice tells me that I am broken for good already. I feel like those cartoon characters with an angel and devil on their shoulders, but I just seem to have a devil and an even meaner devil, and there are hundreds of them. Perhaps Fatima just spotted it early – she saw Satan within me before anyone else could, before I could.

My brain tells me what to do and it is like I don't have a choice. This booming voice tells me I am disgusting and I believe it. I don't have time for friends. I am too busy finding places and times to cut myself and all my energy goes into keeping it a secret. It is my secret. Their conversations seem pointless now anyway. I don't care who likes who or who is good-looking. I don't even notice people when I walk around school. It is just me and these terrifying voices in an empty world. I've almost forgotten about you. I am surviving, so I don't have time to think profound thoughts. I just have to get through each hour and plan my breaks for pain.

I begin to think it is less of a secret. People are noticing. I want everyone to go away; we live in such close proximity. I am about to go to sleep. There is nobody else in my dorm this evening. This is a good thing: no prying eyes and I can keep the light on. A teacher comes in and tells me to move to another room, she doesn't want me sleeping on my own. The following evening, she tells me to go to the health centre. She says that she cannot take responsibility for me any more. I am like a hot potato; nobody wants to be in contact with me for too long. I walk across the school in my pyjamas, carrying my giant Winnie the Pooh bear, to the nurse. I walk past groups of people that I'd spent all of last year trying to impress. The nurse takes me to a white hospital bed with itchy covers. She gives me apple juice and water. She shows me where the emergency button is and hands me a landline phone. I think that the time for emergency buttons has passed. I call you.

"I want to come home now."

I am now more scared of myself than I am of you. I cannot be stuck at this school any more, it is destroying me. You are in London at a friend's house but you stay on the phone. You keep asking why I am in the health centre. We don't really speak; I am struggling to form coherent sentences. I don't understand why I am in the health centre. I don't understand why I am not at home and why I being kept away from you. You stay on the phone until I eventually fall asleep.

DANGEROUS SALVATION

Four days ago, we were the danger, now we – alone – are the salvation. I am promoted from violent mother to mental health nurse. On the train home from London, I speed-read the literature on self-harm, then I put a call through to the GP. I get a call back from the duty doctor who has examined you so that I know what to do when we are reunited.

"As alarming as it looks," he tells me, "it is quite common these days. Keep them clean, offer her alternatives and try not to overreact."

"Alternatives like what?"

"Holding ice …"

In a bowl at the kitchen sink, I dilute the Dettol and roll up your sleeves. The cuts appear fairly superficial but, my God, there are so many of them, criss-crossing your translucent snow-white skin, like striations in marble. I may have appeared matter-of-fact, Roxy, while I doused cotton wool in the milky antiseptic and wiped your arms. But inside, I was bleeding. Even now, I feel pain when I see your scars. It is the pain of a mother failing her daughter. That night, I set up the sofa bed and sleep in your room. You are furious (oh, the irony), oscillating between non-responsive and aggressive. Sometimes you appear so vacant it is like you don't seem to comprehend what is happening or why you have to stay at home. You don't want me anywhere near you, but I am not budging.

The literature and the doctor describe self-harm as an urge. Everyone keeps telling me that it is your prerogative and quite normal these days, that I shouldn't overreact. So I won't. But you are going to have to do it under my watchful eye. Every cut you make, I will be there with the Dettol and cotton wool. I will accept it, but don't ask me to condone it. Dettol is my revenge. Cleaning cuts is the first tangible thing I am able to do. You cut to gain control over your pain. I clean them to gain control over my pain.

You are twitchy even in sleep. You sleep off and on; I know this because I don't. The moment the door moves, you sit up in bed. The perennial light sleeper.

We aren't entirely alone, thankfully, because the next morning at 11 a.m., Freya, the brilliant social worker, comes to see you. Afterwards, I walk her to her car. I will never forget what she says next.

"Roxy is a very, very ill girl," she says, putting her hand on my arm. "No locked doors, do not leave her alone for a minute and if anything happens, anything at all, dial 999 immediately."

She doesn't have to tell me what "anything" means, but 999, really? Are we really there?

"Yes," she confirms, "we are really there. You need to make an urgent referral to a psychiatrist, now." Then she tells me again.

"Dial 999 the moment you think you can't contain this. That is what they are there for: emergencies. This is one."

It is like being handed glasses when you didn't know you had bad eyesight. Or a slap in the face to quieten the hysteria. It stings. Roxy is ill. Perhaps it sounds mad to you that this is news, but it is news. Roxy is a very ill girl. Everything changes after that and the hunt for help begins.

So how do I go about getting an urgent psychiatric referral? We need to be referred to the Child and Adolescent Mental Health Services (CAMHS). And to do that we've got to go back to the GP. I ask the school doctor first, thinking this will be speediest.

"He is not legally obliged to see her now that she is home."

But she only just got home. "You understand this is urgent?"

"He is not legally obliged to see her now that she is home."

"Yes, thank you, you said that."

I phone the GP surgery again and request an emergency appointment. Meanwhile, we wait. Over the next year, we get very good at waiting.

While I have been told not to leave you alone for a minute, I have also been told, in the same sentence, not to be too in-your-face. I find myself waiting around corners, nipping into side rooms, tracking you around the house as you try to get away from my cloying presence while I try to keep you in sight and remain out of sight. Doors open, doors close, tiptoe, track, double back. Every time you go to the loo, I creep up to the door and listen. If you stay in there too long, if it gets too quiet, if you run the tap for too long, I appear as if by magic, having been there all along.

I drag you to the surgery, though you don't understand why you have to go. The doctor is the same doctor you saw when you were at school, the same doctor I spoke to on the phone about cleaning the cuts, the same doctor who has already physically examined you and the same doctor who knows you were sent home because the school couldn't keep you safe. You're right, this is pointless.

He starts asking you questions. It's cack-handed and clumsy. I feel you retreat to a place I cannot reach you – you clam up, go mute. He is unnerved by the way you look at him, so turns to me. I relish that for a brief moment. I know too well how unpleasant it is to be cut down by that laser-like expression. I don't want to answer his questions any more than you do. But I can't opt for silence. Silence doesn't get the referral.

He is tapping things out on his computer. I mean, what the hell is he waiting for? I want to throttle him and stamp my foot, but I can't. It has to be his idea, his diagnosis.

I decide to stare at him with the same expression you are. He looks suitably unnerved. Good. I think I hate him.

"Feels to me like you need an urgent referral to CAMHS to see a psychiatrist."

"Yes. Please. Thank you. How long does it normally take?"

"They should get back to you next week."

I smile dumbly and swallow swear words. We hobble out with a prescription for lorazepam to get us through. Lorazepam, from a family of psychoactive drugs called benzodiazepines. Like Valium, it is addictive, requires increased dosages to reach the same effect after a relatively short period of time, and its side effects mirror the list of uses, it can cause the very thing it is trying to cure. How can I willingly put this stuff in your body? But I do.

*

I leave you at home with your dad. I am taking your sisters to stay with some friends. To give them a break. I do this a lot over the next coming weeks. On the way home, I call.

"Everything okay?'
"Yup. Roxy's having a bath."
"What!" My blood runs cold. "No! She can't. You can't leave her alone." I know you've done this because your dad would never walk into the bathroom even though I have taken the lock off the door. Damn it, I should have seen that coming. I need to stay several chess moves ahead.

"I'll sort it," he says, and rings off. A few minutes later, I get a text from him.

R ok. I'm sitting outside. We're doing a music quiz X

LET ME PEE IN PEACE

The next day, my teacher pulls me out of lessons and walks me into town for a cup of tea. She takes me to a cafe with floral wall-paper, the tea pots are covered in knitted tea cosies. I feel sick. I choose a rose tea and she has a piece of cake. I am expecting a lecture on how she is worried about me, the usual teacher bullshit. But it doesn't come. She asks about my sisters and my dad's work and other mundane things. Even on the walk back, she doesn't even ask if I am okay. As we walk back into school, I realize why she had taken me out. She didn't want to find out if I was okay at all, she wanted me off the premises so they could investigate. This all comes together in my head when I see some of my friends walking out of the head teacher's office. They see me, look at each other, and walk in the opposite direction.

I am made to sit in the waiting room outside the deputy head's offices for what feels like hours. It is like a fish tank. Students walk past, make eye contact with me, and then snigger between themselves. I feel like a part of some sick exhibition – come stare at the slut who has lost her marbles. I don't really care. Stare away. I just need to get to the bathroom. I can feel my blade in my pocket and I run my finger along it. The sharp edge strokes my skin. I cannot wait any more. I go to the bathroom and cut. A wave of relief washes over me. I can breathe, I can do this. I can face whatever is waiting for me when I am eventually called in to that office. I wrap my wrist in toilet paper and gently slide my arm back into my jacket. As I walk out the bathroom, the receptionist walks in. That's odd – there is a staff toilet right next door.

When I am finally called in to the office, the head teacher, head of pastoral care and my house mistress are sitting in a line like an interview panel. I sit down on the single chair opposite them and listen. They found some blood on the floor of the bathroom after I had walked out. They know I have been cutting a lot. They cannot take responsibility for me any more. They cannot keep me safe.

They didn't keep me safe. They refused to fight my battle all those months ago when I first sat in this office. They chose the boys and now they are looking down on this messy girl with such pity. Don't pity me – you helped make this mess of a girl. They don't want another suicide on their conscience, so now they are getting rid of me. They are taking me to the GP so he can clean the cuts and then they are sending me home. They have called my dad. They don't want me to come back for a while. They do not offer me support or any kind of solution. They just hand me over to you so that I am not their problem any more.

The GP is a man. There are so many men. He looks at my wrist and my stomach, but I won't show him my inner thigh. Some things need to be private. His hands are big and cold. I feel so small when he touches me. Dad takes me home and we wait for you to get back from London. We don't talk. Every so often, Dad shuts his eyes and takes a huge sigh. I am a burden. The moment you walk in, there isn't even an inch of empathy. You are angry. I am an Inconvenience. I want to vanish; this is not me. This was never supposed to be my life. You are a straight-to-the-point, no-frills kind of person. This is frills, this is unnecessary drama. This is teenage bullshit that you are not prepared to treat as something real. You sleep in my room and stand outside the bathroom while I pee. You don't do this because you are worried that I'll hurt myself, you do it to a prove a point. You do it to remind me that this is my fault, and what you are giving up to "take care of me".

I hate that you act like I am a nuisance. You don't seem worried at all – I am clearly just annoying you. It is so noisy in my head and you don't understand. They tell me to cut, they make me cut. They speak over each other so I don't understand what they are saying, it is just noisy. I spend a week at home while you treat me like an attention-seeking brat. It feels like you are trying to catch me out, prove that I am faking all of this. God, I wish that I was faking. I watch TV, go on walks, anything to stop my brain forcing me into terrifying places. I cut when I go to the toilet. I say that I am going to take a bath and I tuck my blade into my bra. I shut the door behind me, you are out of the house and I am so relieved to have some privacy. I start to run the bath and I hold the blade in my hand, feeling its power. Dad knocks on the door. I roll my eyes. He tells me that there is a 1980s pop-music quiz in the paper and he would like us to do it together. He sits outside the bathroom door firing questions at me. It is fun. I sit in the water and cut myself while we sing along to U2 together.

SUICIDE WATCH

Every day, we go for walks. They are glacially slow. This one I remember because you lift up the sleeve of your jumper and show me fresh cuts on your arms. It is a heartbreaking sight. They are deeper and longer than the ones from before. There are fewer, but they look more considered, less frenetic, fresh. They are far scarier. I stop myself from putting my hand over my mouth in shock. I want to weep, I want to shake you, make you stop … But I can't do any of those things. Don't overreact. What options do I have? Ice or 999. Without a doubt, 999 scares me more.

"Please don't do that to your beautiful skin any more," I plead. "There are other ways."

"I'll stop," you tell me.

I put my arm around you and once again, we hobble home. Next week is too far away. I make sure the ice tray is full, then call the office of a private psychiatrist and leave details of our plight on the answering service. I am told that messages are regularly checked and someone will get back to me.

"Can I go back to school for rehearsals?" you ask me the following day.

Of course you can't. This naivety poleaxes me. You're not even allowed to go to the loo on your own.

"The school are worried about you," I start tentatively.

"Why?"

Why?! You don't seem able or willing to link the two.

I don't give you a straight answer because I don't have one, so I take advice from the social worker and the counsellor and the school about how to proceed. Everyone agrees, you need a psychiatric assessment and I need to find the words to tell you this. The elephant in the room is now a herd.

We head out for another walk with the dog and it feels like I am walking a tightrope – but the rope is a razor blade. It is not a question of *if* I say the wrong thing, but *when*, so I lay down the ground rules. We can pause the conversation any time.

"I can't help you unless I know what is really going on. What's going on, Roxy? What's happening?"

"I want to go back to school, I want to do the play."

"The school are worried because they can't keep you safe. They need you to see a psychiatrist."

"Why?"

"They need to know you'll be okay."

"So they won't let me back?"

"Not until you've been assessed."

There is that look again. It is as if you don't believe me, like I am punishing you by not allowing you to go back and perform in the musical. Of course I want you to do it. I want you back at school, participating in your life, making new friends, better friends, but you can't pull a pin on a hand grenade, then juggle with it and wonder why everyone has run for cover. The walk gets painfully slow. You can't walk but you can go on stage? How does that work? I'd like to keep on walking, stride out and get away, but I can't.

"We need to turn back. I've got to pick up your sister."

You slow down further. We will be walking backwards if we go any slower. It's a fairly recognizable microaggression: you are telling me you don't want to be alongside me, you are telling me you don't want to hurry for the sake of your sister, you are telling me you are cross because you haven't got what you want. I can't disguise my gnawing frustration, so I decide to walk ahead and let you come in your own time. I hear a yelp. I look around and you have fallen to the ground sobbing. I go back to you.

"What's wrong?" I ask.

"I feel really ill."

That's all you say, over and over. I sit down next to you. Ice or 999? Acting up or cracking up? Have you got something to tell me or is there nothing to tell? I just don't know. Side by side, we stare out over the nature reserve. It's a popular spot, and people walk past us. Even though they glance at us, I choose not to care. What a sorry pair we are. Maybe we're birdwatchers. Having a picnic. You have your head on your knees and I have my arms around you, so probably not. You put up no resistance. It's like the fight has left your body, along with everything else.

I can see a large group of people walking dogs approaching. They see us and stop; there is some chatter and then they very purposefully turn around and walk away from us. Unfortunately, our puppy had seen the dogs and decided to go and play. I can see them trying to send her back and I call for her, but she's run off with the pack. Eventually, I have to leave you and run over to get the dog. Among the dog walkers is Ryan's mother. We both try to shield her from you, but you look around and recognize her. You are mortified. Sometimes I feel the universe is plotting against us. I get you off the ground, but this last humiliation has done you in. I am not exaggerating when I tell you it takes all my strength – both physical and mental – to get you off that path and back to the car. I take most of your weight with my left arm while holding up the right arm that you had wrapped around my waist. It is like walking with a drunk. You just about manage one foot in front of the other, but only just.

The next day, we meet my cousin in a pub to get Reva and have fish and chips. I am amazed how easily you appear to revert to the gossipy, joking teenager she and her children love. They are hanging on your every word. I sit quietly, watching, sipping a glass of wine and wondering which one is the real Roxy. I am grateful for a moment of reprieve, my duty as guard temporarily revoked. I start to relax. Mistake. While talking to my cousin, you yawn and stretch your arms over your head. You have gashes up your left side, to your rib cage. I only see them for a second, but it is enough. In my mind's eye, I can still see them now. My cousin was looking the other way and the kids were playing outside, thank God, but I see them. It is like being punched in the solar plexus. These are deeper, a dark, foreboding red. When you showed me the cuts on your arms, I was foolish enough to take some comfort. You were trusting me with the information, you were admitting to a maladaptive coping strategy, you were asking for help, you had agreed to stop. Or so I thought. But I now know you showed me enough to make me stop looking. I know in my gut these gashes I was not supposed to see. Always so damn canny. I feel really cross that you are still lying to me, or more accurately being so selective with the truth. I realize then that I can't trust you. That was okay when I knew you, but I don't know you any more.

All weekend, I call the switchboard of the psychiatrist and still no one gets back to me. CAMHS don't get back to me. We limp through each 24 hours waiting for the moment in the day when I can give you lorazepam and your brain and body will disconnect for a while, and you will have some peace. It isn't working. Dark thoughts penetrate your sleep. You wake, flustered and scared.

"I can see myself hanging from a tree."

"Every time I close my eyes, I can see someone hanging from the light fitting."

Your dad and I are beside ourselves. On Sunday night, we call 111 and get another emergency doctor's appointment. In the waiting room, you sit on the floor and stare at me with utter loathing and hatred. I try to get inside your head, but the barriers are up. Once again, when we get in the room you don't want to talk. Once again, when I answer the questions you wince at my words. *God, Roxy, you think I want to say these things about you? I don't! I have to.* The doctor tells us our options. Sorry, option. A&E.

That's it. I don't want to go, but I am not sure I have a choice any longer.

"But you should be aware," says the doctor, "that Child and Adolescent Mental Health workers won't be on till morning, and honestly, you may be put on an adult psychiatric ward for the night."

You look terrified. What if I take you, what if you panic, what if you kick off, what if they won't let me stay, what if they section you, what if …?

"Can you keep her safe?"

I don't bloody know. I think so. "Yes," I say.

He prescribes promethazine, a sleep-inducing antihistamine. On the way home, through the overwhelming darkness, I work out why you're so cross with me. I have told you we would get help and I've failed. We pull up at the house and go in. I follow behind you, I follow you upstairs, I follow you to bed. Finally, I have come to accept that I am on suicide watch.

*

We stand on the threshold of CAMHS. Finally. It is the first of several visits to their headquarters in the city. This is the inner sanctum of mental health services, the holy grail. We step through the glass doors and are immediately faced with a bank of wall-mounted shelves with row upon row of terrifying leaflets. Obsessive-compulsive disorder, depression, anxiety, panic and phobias, understanding borderline personality disorder, schizophrenia, bipolar disorder, personality disorder. It is not a welcoming welcome wall. We wait for our appointment. You are sullen, quiet and nervous, biting your nails, pulling slivers of skin off in your teeth, picking and gnawing and fidgeting. I get up from the plastic chair to stretch my legs and walk about a bit. Then I venture out to the pavement, telling you I'm just going to call home. On my way back in, I surreptitiously stuff any pamphlet that might apply into my bag. Nine. I take nine. Inches of literature that promise "help is at hand". At that time, I still believed it was.

Two people approach us and introduce themselves. They are mental health nurses. My heart sinks for two reasons. Firstly, one is male. I know by now that you're not going to speak in front of a man. Secondly, they are nurses, not psychiatrists. In this game of "get an urgent referral", we've got another level to get through.

"This is their job," I try to reassure you. "This is what they are trained to do."

You shoot daggers at me. This is, once again, not the help I promised you.

In fact, it is the male nurse who I watch work his way into your confidence. He is mild, non-judgemental, he is good at his job. He wants you to tell him what happened.

How many bloody times? I think. *Please don't do this to her, it's not fair.*

"I promise you, if you tell us everything, from the beginning, you will never have to say it all again, as it will be on your record," he says, a notebook in hand.

You look mortified.

I am concerned.

They look on, reassuring.

"We know how difficult this is for you," they say as they coax your story out of you.

I say little and I am very proud of you because I can see how crucified you are retelling the story of the photos, the humiliation, the rejection, the bullying, the shame. They are at once sympathetic and appalled that you have been left to shoulder this alone. They ask, like PC Dawson did, whether the school reported the boys. I tell them that they did not. They exchange looks. We limp out to await judgement – has your story been enough to move to the next level of the game?

There is a flaw in the system, of course, I now realize. You can only tell them as much as you know I know and I don't know very much. We go home.

Five days later, we drive back to the city centre. The phone calls and messages, emails and pleas have paid off. We're through to the next level. You will see the child and adolescent psychiatrist for a full assessment. This is a turning point for us. You are scared; you don't want your dad there, but I remind you that we've been promised you will not have to tell your humiliating story again, this is just about answers and help and – I hope, although I don't tell you this – medication.

We walk in. There is an unremarkable man in a grey suit sitting at a cheap brown table on which are no notes. I am not sure what I was expecting, Freud? From the first impression, he does not inspire confidence. In fact, I would go further: he looks out of his depth. I tell myself I am being judgemental and sit on the plastic chair. We all look at him expectantly.

He asks your name and date of birth, which he writes down on the blank piece of lined paper. I start to pray this isn't as bad as it looks.

"So, Roxana, what brings you here today?"

You appear to have been hit. You slump down the wall and land on the floor. Game over.

I would have joined you there, but I don't have that choice. However furious I am in that instant, you must get up, we have to get back in the game. You refuse to speak. Hatred radiates off you. I know this is hard, but we have to do this and obstructing help only harms you. So please, get off the floor and speak to the man. But you won't. Or can't. Either way, it doesn't matter, we have one hour and we're wasting precious minutes. I tell you to go out so I can hurriedly tell our sorry tale without you having to hear it. So we begin. It turns out the man is a locum and he has been told nothing. It's appalling how mismanaged and incompetent the whole sorry event is and, for that reason, it is a turning point. From then on, we go hurtling in the wrong direction for a long, bumpy, painful ride. He prescribes lorazepam and melatonin. There must be something better than this? You and I are deflated and furious, we both want the same thing – help – and I think at this moment we just blame each other for not getting it. Your dad and I have forced you to see this person against your will, all promises broken, and you have failed to help the psychiatrist help you, so we are stuck – none the wiser and no closer to understanding what is going on.

The overall effect of the longed-for meeting is disastrous. We are back to opposite ends of the ring, scowling at one another.

The week limps on. The family limps behind it.

You do the play.

"I've designed a way to hide the cuts," you say. Your costume is a tight black sleeveless dress and you have made two arm sleeves out of tights that are the same colour as your skin tone. I do not know how to respond to this.

Watching you on stage is toe-curling. I don't understand why you would put yourself under the heat of a spotlight when you are hating every second. Your wings are burning, my beautiful moth, and I can't extinguish the flames.

We are on the high street, surrounded by busy stalls and bustling people, but you are making it abundantly clear that you don't want to be with us to watch the Christmas lights to go on. Your sisters are loving it, so I tell you to go back to the car and wait, but your legs give up so I get the car, bundle you in and we go home. However, you're back on stage that night. Forgive me for questioning what is going on. The old doubts are returning. I find myself watching you suspiciously, it seems, and I am no pro, that the moment I get in any way frustrated by your behaviour, it escalates. We are back on the floor – literally and metaphorically – meaning I have to stop, surrender, soften and pick you back up. This makes you dangerously powerful. I am aware you're manipulative. You always have been. I am used to holding firm, but what happens when being strong isn't helping? It feels you are working against yourself – and any act of mine to counter that work is interpreted by you as a direct threat. We are now working directly against each other. Since the terrible meeting with the locum, I am back in enemy territory and under a renewed attack I do not believe I deserve. It pisses me off; I am only human. I know when I am becoming an incendiary element, so I do what some of us are luckily able to do in times of distress: I call my mother.

ON A SCALE OF 1 TO 10

The first people I see from CAMHS are a woman and a man. Why a man? Why are there so many men? This man looks at me and he promises me that if I tell them my story, I will not have to say it to anybody else ever again. I can do this, I can say it out loud one more time. It is all so difficult to say. The photographs are so embarrassing and I want to die as I sit here trying to put these photos into words. I hate the word "nudes", that's not what they were, I don't want to use that word. So I say "these photographs" and they ask what photographs. Don't ask what photographs. They know what photographs. Then there is the running away. It feels like another person ran away, like it wasn't me. Sort of like I was possessed. How can I explain that when I don't understand it at all, when I don't even remember everything?

So I have to say what I did and I cannot explain it, so I sound like a horrible person. I sound like the attention-seeking, dramatic, spoilt brat that you have spent so long thinking I am. It wasn't like that though, I promise you, I was so confused. I sit here and I tell them and I want to cut but instead I chew at my lip and peel the skin around my fingernails and clench my toes until they cramp. I cannot release this horrible pain that I feel spread down my arms, into my wrists and my fingers and into my ankles and into my back. Then it is over and I have said it all and they smile sweetly, trying to show me that they are not judging me for what I have done, but I know that they are judging me and they are just smiling because that is their job. At least I won't have to do this again.

I walk into the psychiatrist appointment a few days later and he asks me what he can do to help. He asks me to tell him from the beginning. What? No. They promised me. They swore it was the last time. I can't speak. The last bit of strength that got me to this appointment has just drained from my body. My legs are too weak to support myself.

He asks me pointless questions that I do not understand. He is reading them off a list, ticking boxes, he doesn't want to help me. He is just following the formula that he is supposed to follow.

How sad do you feel on a scale of 1 to 10?

Do you have energy to go for a walk?

Do you drink enough water?

Do you want to get out of bed in the morning?

Do you want to kill yourself?

How am I supposed to answer these stupid questions? I know the answers I am supposed to give so that he thinks I am fine. I know the answers that I should give if I want to sound dramatic. I want to tell the truth but I cannot answer such complex questions with a yes or no answer without either sounding overdramatic or like I am lying. If I say that I want to kill myself, you will think I am being dramatic and I have no idea where this psychiatrist will put me. If I say that I do not want to kill myself, then I am lying and he won't try to help me. All this is spinning around my head, trying to break through the sound wall of these cackling voices. I can't process everything, so I just stay silent. There are no right answers, so it is best if I don't speak. I cannot think with all these voices shouting at me. Then you are shouting at me. You are so angry that I wasted the appointment with the psychiatrist. You scream and scream and scream. It is the first time that you seem like you care.

The next day, you go off for a "you day" because you are so angry at me. My grandparents look after me. I have a little sweet pot in my bedside table that I have started putting pills in, only paracetamol and ibuprofen at the moment. I know it is pretty pathetic, but it brings me some comfort. They keep telling me that it is safer to have them there. You are still so angry with me about the psychiatrist appointment. This week, I am going into school for the mornings because I want to go back. I cannot sit at home any more. I am feeling better, stronger. I cannot let those boys hold back my life any more. I am behind in lessons. I feel stupid. My head is so noisy that I can't focus on the numbers in maths. The girls on the table behind chatter and chatter and everyone is chattering and it is so loud. I can't join in with any of these conversations and I can't decipher what lots of them are saying.

We are going to this stupid light festival in our town. As we walk down the street, we are stuck behind a group of boys. I realize from the size of one of them that the group includes Dan and Aiden. I am terrified. I feel tiny and in danger. I can't tell you because that would involve mentioning the photos and that is a completely unspoken subject. I seem to have convinced myself that if I don't mention them, eventually you will forget about the awful things I did. I silently beg my sisters to be quieter. I don't want the boys to notice me here. This is too much. It is loud, there are so many people. Everyone shouts everything, nobody just talks. There are teachers and boys all around me. I am breathing quicker and the lights are flashing, making me dizzy. It is so loud and I am scared. You look at me with angry eyes – stop making such a fuss. You don't want me to ruin the event for my sisters, so you take me away.

I am still going to perform in the school musical. I hate every second. I have to wear this tight black dress with a slit up one leg. It shows everything, but everybody has seen everything already. I cut up a pair of pale nude tights and slip the material over my cuts; nobody will know. I hate wiggling my hips to Latin music in front of the school. I hate the watching eyes. I hate sitting backstage, not being able to join in with conversation. The evenings of the play are miserable and humiliating. This voice tells me I have to do the show and I cannot fight it. It tells me that if I don't, then I am the freak that people are talking about. So I do the musical each night, and I cry after as I peel the black dress from my body and the cheap material sticks to the open cuts on my stomach. The other girls admire themselves in the mirror. One whole wall is a mirror. I sit in the corner and look at the wall. Don't look at the mirror.

THE PEOPLE

I have lost faith with the woman who "saved" you the night you ran away because her involvement, as far as I am concerned, has made our situation worse. I have spoken to another therapist, one who comes highly recommended by a trusted source. Now I find myself sinking into her sofa in a small, warm room and feel the tears and fears swell up; glutinous molasses bubbling, always below the surface. What I really want to do is curl up into a ball and tell her that I can't do this any more. Do what, I wonder? Look after my own child. The sense of failure is enormous. I explain the rudimentary facts, which take forever and don't scratch the surface. Naked photos, bullying, social ostracism, self-harm, running away, investigation by social services, purging. I tell her we oscillate between being furious that you treat us so horrendously and terrified that we are still missing something. Talking to her does not make me feel better, it just reminds me how long we've been trying to fix things between us and that whatever I have done, it has not been enough. I just want someone who knows more than me to tell me what to do. My mother sends me an update.

Having a nice day.

How is that possible, I ask the therapist, that you can have a nice day with your grandmother but be so rude and offhand with me? And please, I beg silently to myself, don't tell me she is just a teenager. You've been an extreme teen since you were four. That is the real problem, I tell the therapist – as I told the other therapist, as I tell every therapist – the problem is us. Air crackles with static between us and everyone gets fried. The hour is up and it is time to return. One hour will never be enough time to explain the 90,000 hours that came before this one and have been, for the most part, dominated by you. She has listened, made sympathetic noises in the right places and told me it sounds like I have done a good job in difficult circumstances. She's passed me the tissues. She did say it sounds like you struggle with an inability to read your peer group and that tells her something. I mull this over as I leave. She thinks she can help us; I should make another appointment and bring you this time. I tell her it will be hard to get you through the door, but I make one all the same. Belt. Brace. And anything else that will help hold us up. I check my phone. There is another update from my mother.

No concerns, good form, chatty.

I sit in the car, heart beating hard in my chest, a constant companion, looking at the warm inviting glow of light through the leaded church windows. Inside that church, there is my mother and my daughter wandering around the school Christmas fayre and, according to the text from Mum:

All is well.

Still, I don't want to get out of the car. Truthfully, I'd rather go on driving and arrive at my other life. Any other life.

I enter through thick oak doors with all the good intentions I have gleaned from the therapist: be kind, be supportive, be patient, be brave, be strong and above all things, be consistent. But as soon as you see me, your knees buckle. You don't fall, you stay upright, but you do buckle, and you do make sure I see you buckle. It looks so fake to me that I swear, for a fraction of a second, I almost laugh. Then I realize there is nothing funny about this at all and bristle with irritation while buying some time to figure out what to do next. Why change just because I arrive? I watch surreptitiously and it looks to me that purely for my benefit some physical symptom has to be manifested. You can be fine with your granny but you can't be fine with me because being fine somehow lets me off the hook, and I need to remain firmly on the hook. Which one is the real you? The one who is fine at dinner with your granny or the one with me, stumbling, unable to stay upright? In averting my eyes from you, I find myself standing in front of the headmaster. I recoil from him, sickened with myself for the fake smile and empty greeting I've just given, and I realize this might have not been such a good idea after all. It is really busy and I am horribly conscious that you are surrounded by people who might or might not have seen images of you. I am equally conscious that getting you used to your normal surroundings is what we are trying to achieve.

Always these micro-decisions – based on hastily snatched intel, being made inside fractions of seconds – which then fracture off from all the other options we might've chosen instead, and send us hurtling through time and space. Every single decision. That is what "decide" means: to cut off other options. It is death to an infinite number of possible endings, just as a "homicide" is death of a human and suicide means "death of self". A few laboured steps on towards the beautifully crafted

Christmas wreaths and it is clear to me I've made the wrong decision. It is telling that I can't recall your sisters being there. I can't imagine where they would have been if not with us, so they must have been, but there are empty spaces in the places where your sisters should have been. Your inability to cope with the crowd magnifies. My mother says she's also had enough, so you drive home with her. This is fine by me because the po-faced death stares are hard to take. I am fed up with the roller coaster which only seems to run when I get on board.

I am punished for being a non-believer.

Back at home, you go upstairs on your own and we, trying to carry on as normal, start to make supper. After a while, I ask my mother to go up and check on you. She reappears quite quickly, visibly unsettled. She tells me you are sitting on the floor of your room and when she approached to ask if you were okay, you told her in no uncertain terms to get out of your room. No one talks back to my mother. Minutes tick by. I am nervous, but aware that some kids push when they really want to be held hard, they just don't know how to say it. So I decide to ignore your request to be left alone and go upstairs.

I ease the bedroom door open and find you sitting on the windowsill with your legs hanging out over the edge, staring out into the night. It takes a second to register what I am looking at. The brain runs the algorithms. It is shocking, but I can't shock you. It is frightening, but I mustn't sound frightened. It is alarming, is it meant to alarm? I opt for calm. So, as even toned as a quivering set of vocal cords will allow, I ask you what you are doing.

"The room is too crowded."

I look from the curve of your back, swathed in the cushion of an oversized black puffa jacket, to your empty room.

"They are making too much noise," you mumble.

"Who is, Roxy?"

"The people."

My internal dialogue goes off the scale. *The people? The people? Who are they? What are they saying? How many of them are there?* The knot in my stomach tightens a fraction more. I make the snap decision not to tell you there is no one there. I don't want to disagree with you, it tends to make you angry. Despite the terrifying sight of you sitting on a window ledge, you appear noticeably calm, a child dangling their legs over a bridge, watching a race between twigs, newt-spotting, daydreaming. But this is no daydream, and there is no babbling brook below. Just an uncared-for flowerbed and a weedy gravel path. I don't think you are going to jump out and even if you do – I make a rough calculation about height, weight, distance – you might break your ankles, but you won't die. I replay that moment in my mind later – at any point, you could have tipped yourself out of the window head first and your neck would have snapped in an instant, but I can only operate on the knowledge I had at the time, and at the time, I didn't think of that.

I don't know what to do, so I run and get my mother – the irony is not lost.

Quietly, whispered, hoarsely, so as not to alarm our other daughters. "Mum, come with me, shh, just come with me ..." On the staircase, I tell her that you have climbed out of the window. She can't believe it.

"Roxy says it's crowded in the room."

"I don't understand," says my mother.

"Nor do I. I don't know what to do."

Actually, I know one thing to do. I must tread very, very carefully. We creep back up the stairs so as not to frighten you and make you accidentally fall, which I still don't believe is your intention, but would have been a bloody nightmare to inadvertently cause. Tentatively, we come into your room … I let my mother take over. It is a relief – someone else can make the decision to speak or not speak, touch or not touch, breathe or not breathe. Mum coaxes you in. Honestly, I can't remember what she says. All I know is that I can't speak; it feels like someone has their hands around my throat. You look very lost and very young and so small. My baby girl with the face of a cherub and hair like a Botticelli angel. I have a fleeting but strong sensation that you don't know what you are doing. You slump to the floor, put your head on your knees and stay there. I slide down the radiator next to you and we sit side by side. Quietly, my mother closes the window.

There are moments when you look at me when it appears you do not know me – or worse: what you know of me you neither like nor trust. Your pupils are like pinpricks. You do not want me to be able to see your soul, and I can't. Then you start rocking. I call 111. They suggest A&E. I can't imagine anything worse than taking you in this state to A&E. You are terrified of an empty room; how could I keep you calm in the noisy confusion of an emergency department? Instead, I give you more lorazepam and put you to bed and wait until I know you are asleep.

I go downstairs, pour myself a whisky, sit on the dog's bed with my back to the Aga and let the heat seep through my ribs and into my chest. I calm my nerves and steady myself so that I don't freak your father out. Eventually, I call him in America, where he has had to go for work, but when I hear his voice, I burst into tears.

That is the day I lose you. For a while.

ON THE LEDGE

My granny picks me up today. You have gone to see a counsellor. You are hurting badly enough to get help, but still you think my pain is not real. She takes me to the school Christmas fayre in the evening and we meet you there. It is awful. The festive music jeers at me. Questioning faces look at me – *is she ...? Is that the one who ...? Did you hear what she did?* The lights are too yellow. They swirl around me. My granny tugs at my arm, pulling me back to reality. People are staring at me, like a prisoner who has just been released.

"You shouldn't be here," I hear them hiss.

I know what these people think of me. It is so loud and I find it very hard to smile at people. My smiles are empty now. The simple truth is that even when I am smiling at somebody and they are smiling at me, they are still thinking about what I did, and I want to disappear. I know the stories that these people have been told. They are stories, but they are not what happened. This is what happened: I lost my life. It was taken from me by some bad people. Now they look and whisper and think nothing of it. When I see you walk in, my legs give way. I cannot explain this crazy feeling to you so I show you. I show you and I hope that you have come to rescue me. You are still cold and angry at me for not letting you enjoy the Christmas fayre.

As soon as we get home, I go straight to my room. I am standing in my room and there is nobody there, but it feels so noisy and crowded. I don't know where the noise is coming from, but it is coming from my bedroom and I cannot be here any more. They are all talking and they are all laughing and they are all looking at me and there are so many of them, but there is no them. Who is them? There is nobody there. These voices that have been inside my head before are now everywhere. There are so many voices overlapping that I can't hear what they are saying. They are just talking and I can't breathe. I feel like I am stuck in a lift with hundreds of people, but there is nobody here. I feel so claustrophobic. I cannot find a single place in my bedroom that isn't full of loud, mumbling people. Panting, I open my window and manoeuvre myself so that I am sitting on the sill with my legs hanging out over the garden.

I can breathe and I talk to stars. They don't talk back because they aren't noisy, but they listen. I can still hear the rumbling chatter in the bedroom behind me, but out here nobody is looking and nobody is talking. I look at the ground beneath me and I don't want to jump. I am not thinking profound enough thoughts to think about ending my life. I am just talking to the stars and trying to breathe. My granny walks in and I know what this must look like, but this isn't that. It is just peace. I like the peace. I look down again; this isn't even high up enough for me to die. Unless I dive head first, and then I could do it. But this isn't about that. This is about the stars and the noise and the quiet. I stop looking down and instead, I look out. It is so dark and nobody is looking.

Part 6

GAME FACE

I am driving you back to CAMHS, slowly and steadily, Driving Miss Daisy. Every oncoming car makes you grip the arm rest a little harder. More disconcertingly, you keep checking the seat behind you.

"We should stop," you say.

"I know this is hard, but we need to keep going," I reply. You've agreed this is our only hope. This is key, I can't make you do anything you don't want to do.

"It's not safe."

"It is safe," I try to reassure you.

"They are telling me it's not safe, we have to stop, we have to get out. You need to stop the car."

"We're fine."

We are on a long, straight, single-lane road, surrounded by mature woodland. There is nowhere to stop. I maintain a steady 50mph. Then suddenly, with no warning, you grab the handle and open the door.

"What the f—"

I reach across your body – thank God for seatbelts – jam my arm against your torso and grab for the door.

"It's not safe! We've got to get out!"

Up ahead, I know there is a lay-by in the wood where dog walkers pull in and park, but I worry it is too remote – through your eyes, the trees are spooky, not magical. So with one buttock on the seat, one hand on the wheel, the other hand gripping the passenger-side door handle, we drive on. If I can just get to the houses, I can turn off this road and park up somewhere safe, somewhere far enough away from cars hurtling along a road at 60mph, because my new worry is that you might run into the cars.

213

My bicep is burning. Thankfully, the forestry is thinning, I can see houses up ahead.

"STOP THE CAR!"

"I can't stop here, it's too dangerous."

"I've got to get out, we're not safe!"

You're right, of course, I think, because as I steer the car with one arm, I know for a fact that this really isn't safe. We manifest what we perceive and you perceive danger. What could be more dangerous than you falling out of the car?

"Why aren't you listening to me? They are telling me it's not safe."

"Who?"

"The people."

I decide to talk to them directly. It seems the only option.

"They don't know what they are talking about. I have been driving for years. We will stop up ahead, where it is safe. Then we can get out, but not here."

"Are you sure?" So childlike now.

"Yes, honey."

We pull in and I allow myself to let go of the handle. My arm is burning. Breathe. We both get out of the car, you start to walk back to the road, but I come after you and place myself between you and the smooth tarmac, ready to tackle you to the ground if you make a dash for it. You're eyeing up the road as an option and I wonder what the voices are telling you to do now.

"I can't do this," you say.

Do what? I wonder. *Drive? Go to CAMHS? Live?*

I don't think you know the answer. So I tell you what I have been telling myself.

"We just need to get to this appointment, someone will help us, you'll get the medication you need —"

"Medication?" you ask, looking at me suspiciously. "You think I need medication?"

Your naivety baffles me.

"I don't know what you need, but I do know we have to get there. So when you're ready, we are going to get back in the car." It takes all my powers of persuasion to make you believe me. It is no surprise, therefore, that your faith in me later wanes because everything I promise gets turned into a lie.

I leave you on a chair and walk to the receptionist. She is behind a thick plate of glass. I try very hard to keep the quiver out of my voice. I try so hard that it hurts to speak.

"We were here a week ago," I explain, "and we have an appointment with the Intense Support Team tomorrow, but my daughter has radically deteriorated and I need someone to see her now."

She looks at you, then picks up the phone. I take a seat next to you. I can't remember if I put my arm around you. I should have, but you don't like it when I touch you. In fact, it usually makes you flinch.

The entire front wall of this place is glass. I wonder whose bright idea it was to make the Child and Adolescent Mental Health Services into a giant specimen tank, a constant spectacle of human misery for anyone walking down the street, in case those inside weren't feeling bad enough. There is a girl sitting on one of the bar stools placed intermittently along the glass. Both you and she have your heads bent low, C-shaped humans, too young to be so stooped.

You are agitated because no one comes.

"This is not a good idea," you say, looking at me furiously. "We need to leave. This is not a good place to be."

You stand up. You want to go, so I return to the receptionist. Apparently, the staff are all in a meeting, but they will be out. The place closes at 5 p.m. The clock is ticking. I cannot be palmed off another day. I lose the English politeness. I am not in the business of making friends, I am in the business of getting someone to do their job and help a child's plummeting mental health.

"My daughter is hearing voices, they are telling her it is not safe, she tried to get out of the car while I was driving it, last night I found her on a window ledge, and we need help now, not at the end of a meeting."

Behind me I hear a noise. A door opens, people emerge, and I take matters into my own hands and walk up to them. I recall three women, but there might have been more. They are young. Really young.

"My daughter is hearing voices," I tell them. It seems to be the phrase that unlocks the door so I repeat it.

"She needs help now." I am sorry that once again you have to endure the cruelty of listening to your own demise as I bring them up to speed.

"The lorazepam isn't working, the voices are getting worse. More dangerous."

Two of them stay to help triage the seriousness of the situation – or lack of so that we can be pushed to another day. I am not going to be pushed to another day. They are asking you questions, questions I know you hate. I am trying to deflect them by answering for you, but they have angled their attention on you and now you are in the cross hairs. Your eyes dart about. You stare at me, pleadingly: *Why are you doing this?* I fear you'll buckle under the weight of it. And then you do. One second you are standing in front of them, the next second you are on the floor. Now I think, now, finally someone will do something. But no. What they do is stand around you, in a sort of odd circle, perhaps to shield the public from the reality of what a mental health crisis actually looks like.

You lie in the foetal position in the middle of the reception area, a pitiful yelp emanating from your core. The mental health practitioners continue to stand about, looking down on you. No one is saying anything. I want to yell at them. Instead, I use every ounce of self-control left.

"Are you going to do anything?"

"Roxy, is it?"

I nod.

"Roxy," she says, "do you want to stand up?"

Your pitiful yelp continues.

I wait. I wait. I'm waiting.

"Is this normal?" I finally ask.

"Yes."

And? Are any of you going to explain to me what the fuck is happening to my child? Awkward silence.

No. It seems not. It seems we are just going to continue standing around in a circle staring at the crumpled heap on the floor that is you, or was you, I don't know any more.

"Why aren't you doing anything?!"

They look as paralyzed as you do. Perhaps they aren't allowed to touch you, perhaps there is some insurance protocol I don't understand, or perhaps they just don't know what to do. All these explanations for their inertia depress me, because if they don't know how to help you, or can't, what hope is there? The door through which the utterly ineffectual staff previously emerged opens again and a more senior-looking lady walks towards us. I am crouched down next to you, I've been there long enough to lose circulation in my knees, but I don't know how long that is. Two minutes. Ten? It felt far longer.

The lady breaks the deadlock.

"Let's get you up off the floor," she commands, and as if by magic, you do as she says.

"Let's go into my office," she says and now, as if in a trance, you go.

I push myself to stand and feel the backs of my knees scream in complaint. I walk uncomfortably to the chair you'd been sitting on, fall heavily into it, put my head in my hands and crumple. I don't care who can see. This is what a child and adolescent mental health crisis looks like. A mother pretending to have the answers, then collapsing in secret because she does not. Many times, in many moments, I can recall staring through my fingers, holding my skull, trying to squeeze answers out of an ineffectual brain, tears damning the ducts, a scream lodged in my throat, wide-eyed and terrified.

You and the woman reappear. I don't catch the job title on the woman's lanyard.

"I will call the Early Intervention Team and let them know."

"We've got an appointment with them tomorrow," I say.

"I will ask them to start looking for a bed in a psychiatric ward now."

My heart constricts. This news is what I want but what I don't want to hear.

"If things deteriorate …" she says.

Deteriorate? Holy fuck. How can this get worse?

"… I know, A&E."

We hobble out, and our exit coincides with groups of kids leaving school. They fill the pavement, four or five across. You shuffle slowly alongside me. Some kids laugh.

"Shut up," says a boy, sharply. "Can't you see she's not well?"

I look at him gratefully, then back at you. It's taken this kid seconds to deduce everything. You are not well. That doesn't stop CAMHS jettisoning us out of the door because I suppose you're not "not well" enough.

I decide to stay in the city centre – less travel, less friction, less having to hide this all from your sisters. We find a B&B.

So now what? We opt for a comedy at the cinema, but the opening line of the film, I kid you not, is a girl telling her tutor she wants to kill herself. Not so funny. We leave. You want to go and see trains. Why trains? I don't know, but it's better than the cinema. I decide not to get distracted by why you want to see trains and instead focus my energy on accepting what is. You want to go and see trains and so we will go and see trains. The station is a classic Victorian brick building: high archways, a chilly, echoing space filled with late-evening stragglers, the faint aroma of metallic breaks and diesel, the last hiss of the coffee machine as it is cleaned and switched off for the night. We stand at the glass barrier and watch the tired train huff with resistance. Occasionally a person passes through the barrier and boards. But not us. We wait and watch. Eventually I sit down and leave you to talk to the train. My presence feels like an intrusion and I won't be able to hurry you. Finally the automated announcement informs us that the train waiting on platform 2 will shortly be departing. I can't remember where to. The doors bleep and close, it girds its loins and the last train heaves itself into motion. I am cold to my bones. It is time to go.

"Will I ever see the train again?" You ask in a childlike sing-song voice. It's melodic, but I don't like the tune.

"Will there be another train?" It is now so late that all the trains are gone.

"Why aren't you sad that the train is gone?"

How to answer such questions?

"Even trains have to sleep," I say, nonsensical. But it makes enough sense to you to get you to return to the B&B. Walking is painfully slow. Suddenly this small city feels very large.

"I am going to have a quick shower," I tell you. The hot water is bliss. I turn it way over the recommended click of the thermostat setting. My game face falters when I return to the room. You have taken all the pictures down and turned them to face the wall. I must have looked confused.

"They are saying horrid things to me."

"What are they saying?"

You look at me as if I am an idiot and don't answer the question. I have purchased a quart of whisky, which I pour into my tooth glass and dilute with cold tap water, and we both get into bed. You have lorazepam, I have whisky. Occasionally I look at your precious few pills and feel tempted to pop one myself – two, if I am being honest. I would really like to sleep without one eye open, one ear on and one heart breaking.

The following morning, we eat cold white toast with butter and marmalade while your drama exam takes place without you. From this moment on, a lot of your life will take place without you.

I can see the chevroned brick pattern on the ground of the newly laid pedestrian zone as we inch our way forward through the city centre. Having had time to spare all morning, we now have no time. We cannot be late, and we cannot miss this appointment – it has become everything to me. First you slow, then you stop and then you collapse like a rag doll to the floor, your well-worn black puffa jacket slithering through my hands. I am unable to stop you. The bricks are pockmarked with flattened grey discs of gum, fag butts and pollen dust from a far-off plane tree. I can see and smell the sticky remnants of urine against the wall. Instinctively, I try to get you up; people are now looking at us, but they still hurry by. I see a woman whose daughter you had been with at primary school. I can't immediately recall her name, but we vaguely know each other. She approaches. I am momentarily horrified – why her? Why now? Why someone we know, someone who might gossip? You'll hate it … but then I think, *What does that matter? I need help and help has arrived.*

"Are you alright?"

"Not really." I sound meek and helpless and inexplicably hate myself for it – but in that instant, I *am* both meek and helpless. I need strength and help.

"Oh, okay, well I'll leave you to it …" She speeds away without breaking stride.

Wait! What? Really? I am half holding a kid in my arms who has collapsed on to the filthy pavement and you're walking away? I crouch down and hold you. I don't want you to see her walking away like that. *Slap on the game face, you can do this, Gay.* I feel absolutely alone in that moment. And then, an older man with a friendly smile and a couple of missing teeth approaches.

"Do you need some help?"

The gratitude squeezes my throat like a boa constrictor. I want to tell him we need to get to the Child and Adolescent Mental Health Services, except you cannot walk – but the words don't come out. I can't speak. I try again, but the emotion will erupt and its magnitude is terrifying. Instead, I nod.

He takes your left arm, I take your right and together we raise you off the ground.

"There's a taxi rank round the corner."

I nod again.

"Life is so difficult for these young people," he says.

He looks at you.

"You'll be alright, love. You will."

I try to say thank you, but I still can't bloody speak. He knows; I don't know how he knows, but he knows. You only find true sympathy the hard way. I will forever be grateful that man was there when we needed him most. Another man offers to help, and the three of us get you into a cab. I get in after you, having finally found my voice.

"Thank you, thank you, thank you. I don't know what I would have done if you hadn't stopped, thank you, thank you …" They close the door and I am blindsided by a new sadness. I need them. I can't do this by myself. I'm not strong enough. We pull away and I watch them through the window, my hand to the glass. I feel so sad. I take the memory of the first man's face and his words with me. He told me it would all be alright, that it was difficult for the young, and it was the first time that anyone had said anything positive or sympathetic since this whole horror show started. You talk about him the whole way to CAMHS. His kindness meant the world to us and we clung to it.

The lobby houses a smattering of sad, scarred teenagers sitting on the bar stools with the prerequisite uniform of black clothes. Some have brightly coloured hair, all of them have earbuds jammed in, their nails bitten to the quick, scabbed lips, hunched postures and aggressively defensive, scowling expressions. Then it hits me: these are the kids who are doing well. They've brought themselves here unaccompanied. They are the success stories. We have a such a long way to go to get where they are and they look fucking miserable. The thought creeps in – *What if you'll never be the same again?* – but I bash it down, physically forcing it down my gullet into the maternal magma in my core, where I use it to fuel the fight to get you well. In the absence of sleep, it works well. For a while.

"We are trying to find your daughter a bed."

"Yes."

"There isn't a bed in the city."

"Right?"

"There isn't a bed in the county."

"Right …?"

"There might be a bed in Birmingham." Pause. "Or Manchester."

I must have had a pained expression on my face.

"Probably best to go home, and we will try again tomorrow."

"And what exactly am I supposed to do until then?"

"Keep her safe."

And again, I slap on my game face, swallow the cortisol and walk you out. *I can do this.* I tell myself this as I put you back in the car and drive you home.

MY PEOPLE

I can't see the people, but when I walk down the street I feel them watching me and following me. I know that this sounds like paranoia, but that is not what it feels like. They want to hurt me – but then, I can't say "they" because who are they? There are no people, there is nobody there. So I go around in circles. There is no "they" and there are no people, but I am still so scared.

You take me into the city to stay in a hotel near the CAMHS building. We go to see a film called *The Edge of Seventeen*, but we leave quickly because the main character is sexting, then she is raped in a car and gets very depressed. You are scared, I can feel it. I really don't want to scare you, I'm sorry. They keep telling me to go to the train station. So we go sit by the barriers and watch the trains come in and out and in and out. I am so sad when the trains leave; I want to go with them. They all leave, and I am left sitting here.

There is a picture of a woman on the wall of our hotel room. She keeps talking to me and she is being really mean. It is in her eyes – she is judging me, she thinks that I am disgusting and she tells me that I am disgusting, but her mouth doesn't move. I suppose I know that it is a painting and it isn't a person, but the person in the painting is insulting me. She doesn't like me. She knows what I did, like everybody knows. So I take her off the wall and turn her away from me so I don't have to look at her mean eyes any more. I look at the strip of wire that hangs off the back of the painting, the wire that the picture was hanging off, and the wire isn't mean. I like the wire. It is now quiet and she is not watching me.

I feel like I am being tripped up a lot of the time. People are sticking their feet out in front me. But not people – there are no people. But something is trying to trip me up. I stand at the side of the road and I have this urge to step out in front of the car, just step out in front of the car. It doesn't feel suicidal. I know that is what it sounds like, but it isn't like that. I am not standing here wanting everything to be over, it is just something that I need to do, jump in front of the car. I try to negotiate and pull the tiny part of logical thinking that is left inside of me and I keep myself on the pavement instead. They are trying to pull me, but I stand strong here. This thing inside of me is evil and dark. I sound like a mental person. I mean, I suppose I am a mental person.

THE CUCKOO'S NEST

You wake up scared, as if your nightmares no longer respect the boundaries of sleep. They follow you out of your dreams and contaminate your thoughts. You can see them. I call CAMHS again.

"Still no bed. Well, there is a bed, but not until January."

It's Thursday, the seventh of December.

"It's a busy time of the year."

I am learning that if you take the situation seriously, they take you seriously, so I persist, describing the child on the floor as wide-eyed and manic. Somehow, I have to move you up the list.

She calls back with some good news: the Intensive Support Team who were scheduled to come and see us at home anyway today are in the area. I nearly cry when I realize that the person getting out of the car is someone we have met before: the mental health nurse who first assessed you. I choose to put aside that he had promised you would only have to tell them what had happened to you once, thereby protecting you from having to ever go over the blisteringly painful details of the photographs with people you'd never met.

"So, Roxana, what can I do for you?"

That was then, this is now, and now I need his help more than ever. There is no denying the deterioration in your mental health. You are on the floor, rocking, begging for help. This is no longer a girl burying shame, it is a girl being buried by shame. With them present, and after some discussion, I give you a lorazepam with your Weetabix. That leaves three for the next twenty-four hours. The great thing about benzodiazepines is that they work; the less good thing is that they are highly addictive, mess up your biochemistry and leave you spaced out and vacant. You quite quickly become subdued, curling up on the little two-seater sofa under the window with a blanket and the dog. The team agree that it is no longer possible to keep you safe and it is time for rapid admission. They've been trying, I tell them, to find you a bed. Accessing mental health services is like a grim game of *Super Mario Bros*: there is always another level, you just have to hit the right amount of gold coins. Their visit was like hitting a Power Moon – just like that, we get bumped up the list from emergency to crisis. He puts the call in from our landline, so I know it is real. Once again, I want to weep, this time with gratitude. But once again, I swallow the emotion down – if I started allowing it through, I am not sure I would ever stop. He promises he will ring back with news as soon as he gets back to CAMHS in the city centre.

A couple of hours later, he calls back. I am excited, almost heady. Soon, this will all stop. Not a moment too soon. I tell him the meds are wearing off, you will go from zonked out and zombie-like to agitated and afraid in a matter of minutes, but worse than before. He can hear you in the background. It isn't a human sound, it is a wounded animal, non-verbally communicating a pitiful SOS.

"I've tried everything. I'm so sorry, there's no bed."

"What?"

"We will keep looking."

You howl. You can't be left to be consumed by demons.

"I'm so sorry to tell you this, but I felt I had to report the school to the Child Protection Team."

I am horrified. It was actually one of the few times I did cry. I think it was the shock. Shock of both not getting a bed and now having to deal with the politics of an irate school. We had gone to CAMHS for help, not to make your life worse. And this, I feared, would make your life worse.

"Please don't, I need the school on side."

Why, I ask myself now, was I so weakened by the thought of their authority over your life? Was I ashamed? Or did I want the right to walk back into our old life? If I wanted back in, I couldn't blow up the bridge on the way out, could I?

"I'm sorry, it's already done. Your daughter has been terribly mistreated, the situation has been inappropriately and unprofessionally handled. This is a child protection issue."

That terrific, dedicated mental health nurse was right, of course, I know that now. He was absolutely 100 per cent right. I should have reported them myself.

I feel so sick. Here we are, trying desperately to get you a bed in a psychiatric unit, and they are spending valuable hours on filing a complaint. How does that help you? How does that help me? It doesn't. It just makes me angry – angry that the school hadn't known how to handle the situation, angry with myself that I hadn't known what to ask and so angry with those horrendous, shitty, sexist, manipulative, corrosive, coercive boys. It was spitting, blood-curdling anger and it stayed with me a long time – and none of it was going to help the girl who was curled on the floor pleading for help.

We are left for another 24 hours playing catch-up with the unravelling spool of your mind. All we can do is pray. The following morning, another phone call; a bed has become free. I don't ask how. The mental health nurse is really pleased for us. I can't tell you what a difference it makes to be dealing with one person, with a name, rather than having to explain the situation over and over and over and get nowhere.

"It's a good place," he tells me, "Not that far away. A drive of 90 minutes or so." I don't know if this is miraculous or demonic. The mental health nurse tells me to get there by 3.30 p.m. at the

latest, so we kick into action. What to pack for a secure psychiatric unit? Winnie the Pooh. Check. Fluffy blanket. Check. No
blades. Can't be sure.

"I know what you lot are like," says the young, tautly fit
woman, as she goes through the bag we have just packed as if you
were off on a school trip. "Seen it all before. You'll try anything.
Do you get urges often?"

You are so surprised by the chatty creature, you reply. "Yes."

"Of course you do. See this? This is an alarm. It's attached to
my belt so you can't grab it off me – oh, yes, they've tried, they'll
try anything, but we are well trained, we'll stop you. I'm trained
in all levels of manual restraint, de-escalation skills, breakaway
methods. We're here to keep you safe. You'll be fine, you don't
look like you'll be much trouble ..."

I can't hear the help in that list, I can just hear hindrance. We
are in a red-brick double-storey building surrounded by a wall of
well-trained leylandii and nothing else. Nothing. As far as the eye
can see. Which is far on this flat, homogeneous stretch of acres
and acres of sugar-beet fields. We had begged for this bed, but
now that we are inside this isolated gloomy building, I think, *Run,
run, people, run, let's run!* Even as I walk you in, I want to run out.

But you are nodding and smiling. This is good. I wrapped
my arms around you for the whole drive here, I could feel your
coiled, distressed body straining against mine. I was certain
you would lunge for the door handle, but now you seem to have
relaxed a bit. Are you relieved that someone is finally speaking
your language and normalizing your thoughts? You are smiling
at her. I am encouraged.

The nice, chatty guard continues.

"You will be registered and then assessed by the psychiatrist,
who will go over your notes and medications. Then we will go

through all your belongings with you to check for contraband goods and items."

I think about the contraband list I read on the website and hope you haven't tried anything stupid. Obviously, you've been cutting yourself, and I know how because one fine afternoon when you were out with your dad, I searched through your belongings until I found what I was looking for. You'd taken the smallest screw bit from my drill set and used it to separate the blades from several small, brightly coloured plastic pencil sharpeners. You hid them all together in the bottom section of a small pink girly jewellery box. The blades and screw bit still lie alongside a teething ring you've kept from infancy. Of course, I had wanted to take them when I found them, but I had been advised by the social worker and doctor alike that you would only find more, so it was better to leave them nesting in pink suede and instead, keep telling you how best to keep the wounds clean and avoid infection. Like the teething ring, the blades were how you self-soothed. Unlike the teething ring, they left scars. Wounds heal, but scars remain, striations of white-hot pain stay etched into your milk-white skin.

"She wants to get well," I say, but my voice sounds strangled. "She wants help." I feel like someone has their fingers digging into my throat as I fight to sound "normal".

"Course she does."

"They said something about a teacher being on site, lessons?"

"Yes, the clients come in here to work. They can keep up with their work. You'll see how you feel about that after the doctor has assessed you." In some training manual it must be recommended the patients are called clients. It is to avoid dehumanization. I look at all the security and wonder if "inmate" wouldn't be a better description. So far we haven't seen a member of the medical team.

By the time we do it is nearly 5 p.m. The psychiatrist is Polish, I think – certainly she has a strong eastern European accent. A clever lady, no doubt, but rushed. I hadn't realized the 3.30 p.m. arrival was a prerequisite to seeing a professional member of the medical staff. We shouldn't have stopped to say goodbye to a couple of the DofE girls who'd started to step up and offer support – maybe even friendship. Vital friendship, as far as I am concerned. We shouldn't have stopped at the superstore on the way to buy a dressing gown. The psychiatrist rushes through the drugs, rushes through the voices and visions and tells us not to worry since she will be back the following day to see you properly. By then, she says, you will have had time to settle in. I do not want you to settle in. She assures me that the staff are well trained and will take good care of you.

"She'll be fine."

We are being hurried out, I know it. It's now gone 5 p.m., and it is time for this overworked human to go home. I don't blame her, but I need her, I need her to quell the growing fear that this has turned out to be a terrible mistake.

"She'll be fine." She checks the drugs list again. "We will give her promethazine on top of the lorazepam."

This is the chemical way of restraining agitated and possibly violent children. Sedation, emotional castration. Talk about a blunt object. When are we going to get drugs that cure? What even are those drugs?

The nice, chatty staff member takes you upstairs to go through the things you've brought from home. We'd done a hurried internet search about what to bring. The website had said to bring things to remind you of home: furry cushions, comfy clothes, slippers, notebooks, diaries. It also listed what not to bring. No belts, no sharp objects, no blades, no Pringles ... yes, no Pringles – the metallic lining can be pulled out to form a basic but effective blade. In our new world, a tube of crisps is a weapon, paintings talk and humans howl.

Your dad and I face one another alone. The façade crumbles immediately.

"We can't leave her here!" your dad says to me. Tears are filling his eyes. "What are we doing? How has this happened?"

He's right. How can we be admitting our wonderful, smart, complicated, complex, clever, gifted, beautiful girl into a psychiatric hospital? The computer cannot compute. I can feel myself glitching under the stress of the previous three months.

"At least it is voluntary," I say to reassure my lost and terrified husband. We are voluntarily locking our daughter up. Your dad crumbles because that sounds worse.

"She begged for help," I remind him. This is what the best kind of help looks like. The social worker, the mental health nurse, the therapist, I remind him, all said admission is what she needs and it's a damn sight better than being on an adult psych ward in a huge hospital.

"This is a good place, one of the best."

I am calming him and convincing myself.

It is for kids only; it is small. We are lucky. I mentally brush off the findings of the inspection report I had furtively read while manically packing. Rated: good (safe, caring, responsive, well-led). Requires improvement: effectiveness. What is a unit for if not effectiveness? I guess we will find out.

"We can't go on the way we were," I say. "Remember the girl on the floor, rocking, listening to the destructive voices of people we can't see?"

He nods.

"We are not qualified." It is true, we're not. "This is the best place for her." We keep telling ourselves this.

231

I ask the receptionist how long you are likely to stay.

"Between six weeks and six months. Usually."

"What?!"

"Six weeks is the minimum, six months is the average."

"What about Christmas?"

"Some of the patients go home for the day, but not all."

We go back to the waiting room and not for the first or last time, have to hold our nerve.

A new person appears and instinctively I don't like her as much as the other one. This is only because she isn't the one we have come to know, even briefly, but when you do not know a single face, the one you do know means something. She tells us you're on one-to-one care, which means she will stay with you until her shift ends. Then another carer will take over. When the bedrooms are unlocked, you will be accompanied and when you go to bed, you will be watched. All night. My heart is beating faster.

Your return marks our cue to leave. I try to hug you, but you've become stiff and wary. As we hand you over to this new person, I think it is dawning on you that we will walk out of here and you won't. Can't. You look so frightened. I want to go and I want to stay. I need to leave you but I want to take you with me. I am so confused and scared. I try and get it together so that I can at least appear calm and confident to you so that you feel in safe and capable hands.

"Bye, my angel."

You are led to the double-locked door, through which we cannot follow. You turn.

"I can't believe you're leaving me here ..." Venom. Your eyes are filled with pure venom.

You are whisked through the first set of doors. The second set of doors is released by fobs attached to humans attached to alarms attached to staff trained to restrain.

I grab your dad. Walking back to the car, I find I can't breathe. He gets me into the car.

We cannot face going home, I can't "game face" my way through your sisters' bedtime. My friend who is with them tells me not to worry, to take as long as I need. So we drive to a pub in the next village and sit in a nook, hidden from view. We drink Guinness and cry and cry and cry. Six weeks to six months, and a day out for Christmas. Once again, the insidious, repetitive, cruel, accusatory, angry thought goes round and round: How, how, how, how has it come to this – that we have left our baby locked up, alone, scared, in the grip of a psychotic breakdown? I drink too much to drive, so we leave our beaten-up old Land Rover in the pub car park. I thought I would collect it the next day. It sat there for two months.

CANDY CRUSH ON ONE-TO-ONE

I don't know how many pairs of pants I need to pack. Do I need to take enough for a week? A month? Six months? Maybe they don't have a washing machine. I'm not sure if I need to take my normal clothes, maybe I just need trackies – or they might have some sort of hospital clothing. I'll just take a pair of jeans, trackies, leggings and two jumpers. I've never been very good at dealing with the unknown. I don't know what to do about Winnie the Pooh either; I'm not sure if I'll be able to sleep without him, but the other people there might tease me. I kiss Pooh on the head and leave him sitting on my bed. When I get in the car, I realize that I've forgotten my toothbrush and pyjamas. I just look out of the window.

I think that this is the first time I properly realize that I am totally and completely out of control. Before, I was sort of telling myself that I could switch this off and go back to normal if I really, really had to. That although the voices were winning, if worst came to worst, I could put myself back in control. I want help. I think I know now that I need help, but I am scared. We stop off at Sainsbury's to get the things that I need, but none of us know what I need, so we just walk aimlessly up and down the aisles. When we arrive, you leave and a lady takes me up to my room. She looks only a few years older than me. My room has a bed, a shower and a loo. There is one small window with bars on it. The lady who walked me in sits down and starts going through my bag. She confiscates my belt, takes out the laces from my shoes, she takes away my diary because it has a metal spine and she takes away my school folders because of the metal clip. Eventually she finds the floral pouch with the blades. I had wrapped it up in clothes in an attempt to hide it. When she takes it, an emptiness scrapes through me. My secret power is gone.

"Why are you here?"

I can't speak, but I swear you aren't meant to ask that in these kinds of places – prisons and hospitals and stuff. I don't know what to say. Because I am so sad that I can't do it any more? Because I've gone crazy? I don't say anything.

I have a 10-minute conversation with a psychiatrist who gives me Valium. I feel like I am sleepwalking; this is quite a good thing really – it all just feels like a bad dream. She says that I am on "one-to-one", which means that I have to have a member of staff an arm's length away from me at all times. There are six other kids there, two boys and four girls. They make my cuts look pathetic, they have purple wounds laddered up their legs and arms and they are proud of them. I am the only person for whom this is my first hospital admission. They ask me if I have managed to smuggle a blade or any contraband in. I shake my head.

"Don't worry, we'll share ours."

One of the girls is blonde, with chubby cheeks like a bunny, but the rest of her body is a skeleton. I can see the bones in her fingers, and her knees wobble when she stands up. She has been here for six months and is about to be moved, as that is the maximum time you can stay here. I hold my breath when she walks down the corridor; it looks like she might snap in half at any second. The girl who has the worst cuts and a bandage around her wrist has been admitted from A&E for her third suicide attempt. She is 13. Part of me is thinking how awful it is that a 13-year-old can be that unhappy; surely, she hasn't lived long enough to be that sad. And I am ashamed to say that the other part of me is thinking that if she really wanted to kill herself, she would have succeeded by now.

Jordan is on four-to-one. The problem with Jordan is that he keeps trying to steal the staff keys. Apparently, he succeeded once, so now he has to be circled all the time. We are all sitting in the living room and the phone rings. I stare at it, praying that it's you.

"Hi, yes, I'll pass you over to her."

She tries to pass the phone over to a petite girl who looks about 12, mouthing that it is her mum on the phone. This girl smiles and giggles all the time. She shakes her head, still smiling sweetly.

"Tell her I'm in the shower."

My blades have gone and I need a new secret power. At dinner, I can't eat and I can't drink. It helps that oil pours out of the fish and chips, and the girl next to me says that they've had this meal four times already this week. If strangers are going to send me here and my parents are going to leave me here and these people are going to keep me here, then I am going to have full control over what goes into my body. We are told to go and get ready for bed and I am escorted into my room. I need to pee and wash away the smell of grease. The lady with me insists on coming in.

"I can't be seen naked. Please." *Too many people have seen me already.*

"I'll face the wall."

"Please. I will speak to you the entire time. If I stop for more than five seconds, then you can come straight in."

She relents. First I say the alphabet out loud twice and then the months of the year. I repeat the process until I have washed, but I don't feel clean. I don't sleep at all the whole night. I have to have somebody sitting a metre away from my bed, and this person changes every hour. They play *Candy Crush* for hours. I spend the night curled up, hugging my knees into my chest, willing myself not to cry. I am not homesick, I am not homesick, I am strong, I am not crazy. The people are still here, of course they are, they follow me everywhere. They are watching me and shouting things at me, trying to get me to scream. I will not scream. If I scream, the lady sitting on the floor will hold me down and try to control me – I've seen them do it to Jordan. I am not crazy. I will not cry and I will not scream. I am not sad and I am not scared. All through the night, there is shouting and banging coming from other rooms. An alarm goes off every couple of hours. I am not entirely sure how much of the screaming and shouting is coming from my people and how much is coming from the other patients.

Bang, scream, bang, scream, bang, bang, scream.

I miss the time when it was just one powerful voice in my head, and we argued and we battled and we negotiated.

Sometimes I won and sometimes the voice won, but now there are so many voices coming from so many different places. It is terrifying.

BREAK OUT THE BROKEN

"You do realize she might not see you," says the member of staff as she shows us through to a small waiting room.

"We've been warned," I say.

"Or she might beg you to take her with you."

"We understand that under no circumstances is that happening. We've been told that too."

She's shaking her head, unimpressed that we've come despite the dire warnings.

"We promised her we would bring her some food," I say. Food, ever our Trojan Horse.

She relents. "I'll let the staff know you're here. Something to drink? Tea?"

I nod gratefully and suppress tears. The offer of a cup of tea makes me cry. This morning, I couldn't get out of bed. A boulder pinned me to the mattress and tears leaked out of me. So I'm doing pretty well, all things considered. It's not surprising I'm teary; we've been on high alert for 22 days and nights and then locked you up and left you when we could no longer cope. That's how it feels to me. You are here because we couldn't handle it. I am crippled by fear and guilt in equal measures. So yes, right now, kindness makes me cry.

An orderly brings us tea on a tray, a pot, two white cups, a jug of milk, sugar.

"She's a lovely girl," she says. "No trouble."

The tea and biscuits have gone when a mental health worker comes in and offer us an update.

"She's been very quiet and kept to herself. It is very early days."

"How does she seem to you?"

"Fine."

"Fine?"

"She's not ready to talk yet and that's fine. She's only just arrived. She's no trouble. Very polite."

I have heard this your whole life. No trouble. Very polite. The bolshiness and bad behaviour are very much reserved for me.

"Just one thing we are keeping an eye on: she hasn't had anything to eat or drink."

"What, nothing?"

"No."

"Not even water?"

"Not even water."

"For how long?"

"Since she got here."

The woman leaves. Your dad and I stare at one another. *Twenty-four hours with no food or drink?*

When you arrive, you appear suspicious and guarded, lunar pale. You keep your back to the wall, as far away from us as the small room allows. I step towards you for a hug and you flinch, so I retreat. I have no right to force affection on you. You bristle with fury.

"Why are you here?"

"We wanted to check you were okay."

It sounded asinine as soon as the words were out of my mouth.

"I'm fine, you can go now."

Your dad steps in. "Are people nice, being helpful?"

The fury surges inside you and explodes. "It is shit. A con."

"What do you mean?"

"There's no help, we're just locked up."

"Haven't you seen anyone?"

"No."

"What about the staff?"

"All they do is stop people from hurting themselves."

"Have you seen a doctor?"

"No."

"Therapist?"

"No."

Each monosyllabic answer is spat with force and fury. There is an awkward silence. I know both your dad and I are racking our brains trying to come up with safe ways to get you talking.

"What have you been doing?"

"Nothing. Reading."

"Anything else?"

"No. There is nothing to do. No one does anything here. We're locked into a room all together. That's it."

It sounds desperately unproductive – but I don't know, perhaps you're exaggerating.

"Did you sleep?"

"No."

Pause.

"Someone was sitting next to me the whole night."

"Really?"

"Yes, that's what one-to-one means. Some random person sitting, watching you sleep, playing *Candy Crush*. It's horrendous and they are so loud when they change over shifts, so no, I haven't slept at all."

"How often do they change?"

"Every hour."

I can't help wondering who could stay up all night watching another person's child sleep. I'm in awe, humbled and grateful. I know they are doing the job I feel incapable of continuing to do.

"What are the other kids like?"

"Alright," you soften a bit. "I am the only person in for the first time."

"What does that mean?"

"I'm the only first-timer."

We look on dumbly. You relent.

"The first question anyone asks me is how many units I've done. Which other units I've done."

We catch on slowly.

"This is their second or third time in a unit. One guy has been here for six months and he's not allowed to go home for Christmas!"

I can hear the panic behind the anger.

"All they want to know is if I've brought anything in."

"Like what?"

"Anything sharp. I told them they've taken everything. They're sweet, though. Said it was okay, they'll share what they have."

We are interrupted by another contraband check. You and the member of staff go off together to go through all the new stuff that we've brought you. I turn to your dad.

"We've got to get her out of here."

Of this I am 100 per cent certain. The daughter who wanted help yesterday was still in there – and as angry as she was, and she was burning up with rage, she still wanted to tell us what was going on. It may be dripping in bravado, disguised as hate, but I could just make out the faint cry for help. I did not think that would be the case on Monday. We take her or we lose her. I know it with every molecule of my body. I can still feel it. Moments of certainty are rare in life, especially when it comes to parenting, but I was absolutely certain about this. Your dad looks at me, terrified and barely able to speak, holding his hand over his mouth, holding back the tears and panic, but I know I am right. Just about this one thing, I know I am right.

I am tough, tough enough to leave you there if that is what you need. But I feel in my waters, in my core, that this is not what you need. I tell your dad to let me do the talking. He nods, acquiescing in a manner I have never seen before nor since.

I go and find the psychotherapist and ask why you've not seen anyone.

"The trouble is you arrived late yesterday, so Roxy couldn't have the full assessment." I note her Canadian accent.

We were 15 minutes late, but I'm not going to pick a fight with this lady.

"What about today?" I ask.

"She doesn't come in on Fridays."

I just let that hang.

"Since there are no therapeutic sessions over the weekend, do you think we can take her home?"

"That's not usually allowed."

"The main purpose to stay here is to keep her safe, but we've been doing that for days, I know I can do it at home."

"Is she sectioned?"

"No, she came voluntarily because she really wants help, but I can feel that is changing. She's pulling away. She's not eating or drinking. That is a protest, but at home she'll get good food, see her dog, feel safe."

I know I can do it. I'd had a day without you and it was not a day I wanted to repeat. I am stronger than I realized. I can feel the woman wavering. Thank God you've been so bloody well behaved. You are stronger than you realize, too. I push a little harder.

"By Monday, we might have missed the window where she is complicit in her own recovery. She came here to get help and she's not getting it."

The clinician looks at your notes again. "She's off one-to-one already …" I can see her tumbling the thought around in her head.

"I will sleep with her. We'll walk the dog. And on Monday, when the therapeutic staff and activities resume, I will bring her back."

"I do see your point. She's not hurt herself or anyone else." She studies me. "As long as it is only for the weekend."

"Absolutely."

"And you bring her back on Monday."

"Absolutely."

I don't punch the air, but I want to. Instead, I sign a release form that states officially, in ink, that I am removing you from the facility *against medical advice*. The signature protects them. Not you. If you kill yourself, it is on me. I weigh this up. The reality is that whether you are locked up here or home with us, it is on me as your mother, us as your parents, it is all on us. It is a long, lonely road. I am so thankful that your dad and I have each other. I know we do things differently, we are different people, but mostly we know when to use one another's strengths. Today is the day to use mine.

You come back downstairs.

"You're being allowed home for the weekend," we tell you.

Your reaction is one of pure emotional release. You cry and sort of try to climb back up the armchair. Further away from me, us, the tea tray.

"You can't do that, you can't make me come here and then tell me I can come home, you can't just do that. Just when I've got my head around this, it's not fair."

I should have seen this coming; you've always had a problem with transition. You are panicking now. If this isn't the place to get me better, where is?

"It's just till Monday. There is no help till then anyway, you'll be stuck in that room, reading, so you may as well come home. Daddy will cook. You can see the dog. The therapist is happy to let you come home. She thinks it is a good idea."

It percolates, then suddenly hits the mark – it is real, it isn't a trick, you can walk out of the previously locked door. I think that option was intoxicating in a way, it was like you'd been holding your breath and now you could breathe. You lunge forward, grab the milk jug and drink its contents.

That is when I know we are definitely doing the right thing.

We are bustling you out like a celebrity through the back door. But we are not quick enough. We are surrounded by kids patting you on the back. I notice the unhealthy pallor of incarceration.

"Bye, Roxy."

"Lucky you, Roxy, going home."

"Have fun, Roxy."

One boy uses the distraction to run into a wall. The atmosphere tenses up, and everyone has to go back behind the second door. Staff with alarms move past us with purpose. The Canadian psychotherapist corrals her herd brilliantly towards the self-locking door with safety glass. The air prickles for a moment, then back the clients go, waving and smiling. Sort of smiling. The girls have tragically terrible teeth.

The calm, competent staff member who checked us in yesterday now checks us out. I start to explain my reasoning to her. She is a little less cheery and she has no time for my drivel.

"Just make sure you come back on Monday."

It's a warning and she is right to make it. An empty bed is a wasted bed; the list is too long and the need too great. But for that moment, I am as selfish a human being as I have ever been, and I choose the needs of my child over another. I am not entirely sure that was why there is an edge in her voice, though. Either she doesn't like the shift in the power dynamic, or she thinks I am soft and you are spoilt, and she has no respect for either. This impressive, dedicated young front-line carer spends her days outfoxing the foxes. She recognizes a ruse before it is fully thought through, and that Friday afternoon, she knew what I knew.

Walking across the car park towards our car, I half expect a hand on my shoulder. I have convinced the therapist of my intentions to return, but not your guard. She is too wily for that and always on alert for the hidden Pringle foil. I get you into the car, climb in next to you and tell your dad to drive. I have just lied to bust you out of a secure medical facility, with no intention of ever taking you back.

Your dad puts his foot to the floor and you start talking, non-stop, while inhaling ham.

"They all wanted to know how many units I'd been to before, I didn't understand what they meant, I was the only one who was a first-timer, some had been in three, four times, one boy had been in there six months already and wasn't being allowed home for Christmas, I just sat on the floor and read, we were locked in to one room all day, there was no lesson, they were sweet, the girls, they wanted to know if I had smuggled anything in, they said they had ways, that they would share what they had, they ate Pot Noodles, there was a boy who ran into the wall all the time, there was a boy who threw himself down the stairs, the staff sat next to my bed, every hour they would change, I woke up every hour that they changed …"

The words tumble out of you, breathless and urgent.

"Am I going back, am I going back, am I going back?"

I think it best to tell you the truth. "No. We will go to London and get outpatient help there."

"But what about the rest of my stuff?"

"We'll get your stuff," I tell you. We never do. There was never the time nor the inclination to return.

We get you home and put you on the sofa, under a blanket in front of the telly. I silently creep upstairs, open the pink suede jewellery box, there is one bright yellow sharpener with its blade intact. I take it and the tiny screwdriver. You will be under constant surveillance, so if you want to cut yourself, you are going to have to go through the trouble of finding a new blade. I wonder if you notice the kitchen knives are missing.

I go to my computer and see that three emails have come in from your school.

The first is from the deputy head.

We have been managing some very concerned and tearful close friends of Roxy, who had been frightened by her level of anxiety and distress. Bearing this in mind, we would be extremely grateful if you would not contact Roxy's friends for the time being.

A three-minute farewell to remind you that despite everything you are going through and everything you continue to face; you have friends to come back to. Three minutes to hug two girls goodbye.

The next email is from your tutor.

Subject: Super Report!

You receive a wonderful end-of-term report. He describes this feat as amazing, and amazing it is. He wishes you well and hopes to see you back in school at the earliest opportunity. The deputy head wishes to brush you under the carpet like a sordid little mess. Thank God he's not head of pastoral care, except – shit, he is.

Then the proverbial straw for the day, 9 December 2016.

Subject: School Release Song for Charity

They have produced a song to raise money for the school's charity of the year, Young Minds. I will repeat that, the school's charity of the year – Young Minds. The charity's mission is spelled out on their website: to make sure young people struggling with their mental health get the best support possible. *Support.* I believe the girls who produced that song have pure intentions. Sad that the school – the very school with posters for Young Minds *everywhere* – couldn't stick to the same song sheet.

The school took my A-grade girl and broke her.

RED LEATHER BELT

Today I don't eat breakfast. Ha, I am in control. We are all taken into a room with chairs arranged in a circle. We all have to say something we like about the person sitting to our left. When it gets to the girl sitting to the right of me, she runs out of the room crying and a member of staff goes after her. I decide not to take it personally. Ten seconds later, an alarm goes off and four more members of staff run out of the room. It turns out that the girl had been pulling staples out of the wall display and had tried to hide them in her bra – that afternoon the staples are replaced with Blu Tack.

Every door can only be opened by a member of staff, and you can't go into a room unless you are supervised, and you can't be in your bedroom during the day. The problem is that there are barely any staff, and Jordan requires most of them, so none of us can go into any of the rooms because there is nobody to supervise us. I am sitting on the floor of the corridor with my back against the wall and my legs stretched out. I have been here since breakfast, which was three hours ago. Another patient asks me why I am in the hospital; I still have no idea what to say. Everybody else has announced that they have an eating disorder or anxiety or depression or they are suicidal or they have multiple personality disorder. They have made fun of people who see things and hear things, the "crazy people", they say.

"You aren't a psycho, are you?" a girl hisses at me.

"No, of course not."

They laugh with relief. I am too messed up even for a psychiatric hospital. The girl opposite me has tried to hack into her arteries three times, and I am the one who is crazy?

At lunch, the topic of conversation is Christmas. I don't eat or drink. Ha. They have decided which of us will be allowed to go home and which of us will not. I am told that I haven't been here long enough for them to have decided and they will let me know. Everybody else is told that they can go home for two nights and return on Boxing Day; their parents will have to supervise them constantly and if they try to hurt themselves in any way, then they will be sent back. This is everybody apart from Jordan. Jordan will have to stay in the hospital for Christmas with three members of staff. They say he can choose what they have for Christmas dinner and one present under £10. He asks for an Xbox and turkey. They say he can have a pencil case and pizza.

We go back to the corridor floor and wait for Jordan to do the next crazy thing. He punches one of the members of staff and gives her a bleeding nose. The girls laugh for half an hour; it

247

is a much-needed source of entertainment. To distract us, they bring out a bowl of what looks like watery cake mix and tell me to stick my hand in it. It is rock solid; however hard I push, I can't get my hand through the surface. When I take my hand away, it looks like liquid again. It is a mixture of cornflour and water, which is a liquid but becomes a solid when pressure is applied. It entertains us all for 45 minutes.

Nobody working here knows my name, they just address me as "you" or "the quiet one". I ask to go up to my room to get my book, and they tease me for reading on the weekend and being a nerd. When I stand up to walk, the dining room spins around me and I feel like I'm going to be sick. I grab on to the wall to stabilize myself. Walking down the corridor, my legs suddenly feel like string – they will not stay rigid. My legs give way and I fall to the floor. I just lie there. My whole body feels like jelly. I am weak and tired. I stare up at the white lights above me and the prickly carpet scratches my neck. I hear an alarm ring and then there are three faces staring down at me. One lady sits me up, holds my mouth open and pours apple juice into it. I spit it out.

"If you don't swallow the apple juice, then you will be shut in a room for every meal and you won't be allowed to leave until you have eaten all the food."

I swallow the apple juice.

They move us all into the dining room and I position myself in the corner. The people are everywhere – they jeer at me, teasing me, trying to get me to respond – but I am determined to not let anyone at the hospital know how messed up I am. I focus on my book, I imagine a little man running along each letter, sliding on the loop-the-loop of the letter "e". I hide myself in *The Perks of Being a Wallflower*. I read the book from start to finish yesterday evening, but it's the only book I have, so I am reading it again.

The girls are having a competition about who has done the worst things to themselves and who has had the worst things done to them. One girl is about to be moved to another treatment centre and she is showing off the information pack. The booklet has dolphins on the front and smiling children hugging each other. She very loudly instructs nobody in particular to remind the new facility that she cannot be touched or handled by men due to past experiences.

The building has a nice garden with a tree and a swing. I ask the girl who has been here six months when we are allowed to go outside. She says that she hasn't been outside since she got here. The whole room begins to shrink, the walls move closer to me and Jordan's shouting gets louder. I can't be here. After every page I read, I look out of the window to check if you have arrived. You said you would be here at 3:00, and it's 3:15. You aren't coming. You got home and realized how much nicer and calmer it is when I am not there and now you aren't coming back. I am stuck here, and nobody is doing anything to help me get better. I realize that they are just trying to keep us alive, none of us are ever going to get better. But also, I am safe. Nobody is trying to hurt me, nobody is asking me lots of questions. Maybe I am happy here. Nobody knows me and nobody cares what I've done and nobody whispers about me.

Five minutes later, your car speeds into the car park. I can't speak to you or look at you. I don't know what to say. I can't possibly explain this place to you, it would be like trying to explain human life to an alien. Nothing in here is anything like what is out there. You have brought me a bag of food, like mozzarella and Parma ham. I don't take it. Ha, I am in control. You've also brought me a bag of stuff. We sit in this tiny room with three purple chairs. I answer your questions, there is so much I want to tell you, but I feel like I can't speak. How do I tell you that I haven't been into any of the rooms they told us about when we arrived: the therapy room, the living room, the education room? I feel safe here. After a while, they tell me to bring the bag of stuff to my room so they can check for contraband, and I leave you sitting on the purple chairs.

Half an hour later, I am told to pack a rucksack, as I am going home for the weekend and I will come back on Monday. I don't want to go. Everybody keeps telling me things and sending me places and now that I am here, they want me to go. I don't want to go home for the weekend; nobody else is going home. I don't understand. Nobody told me that I was going to come and go and come and go. I pack a small bag with one outfit, my new toothbrush and I ask them to get my diary from contraband. When a member of staff opens the door to the lobby where you are waiting, the other kids throw themselves out of it trying to escape. I stand with you, looking back at the door. There is a pyramid of children. Three girls are sprawled across the floor, trying to army crawl their way through the staff's legs. Jordan is trying to force his way through the wall of staff members as he flails his arms around. The girls' faces are lit up with gleaming smiles and some are giggling. They all know they can't escape, but it's fun to try. I get it. I smile and laugh too. You and Dad look terrified, like they are a pack of lions trying to break out of a zoo – but they are just kids. We are all just kids, wondering how we ended up being so messy. When I step outside, the fresh air whirls around me and pierces my lungs, but it feels good. I devour a pack of Parma ham like a bird of prey ripping at a carcass. I think part of me knows that I am never going to go back to the unit. I am sad because my favourite jeans are sitting in contraband, with the red leather belt that I got for my birthday and all of my shoelaces. I am scared because even though I am free, I am right back at the beginning.

*

We are on a dark train platform and it is raining. I clutch on to Winnie the Pooh and will my brain not to take me back to the hospital. I can't think about Jordan or *Candy Crush* or the bars on the window or the fish and chips or the apple juice. Instead, I think about my favourite red leather belt that is still sitting alone in contraband.

The past few weeks, you have talked non-stop about getting a bed in a hospital. Now I am out of hospital, but everything is still so loud. So what do I do now?

I am comforted by the arrival of the train.

THE LONG ROAD TO RISPERIDONE

Leaving you in the waiting room with your book, I enter Dr V's office alone. I'm learning on the job. You hearing – or worse, you having to retell – your story is an automatic setback. I have elected to do this with you as an outpatient in London, so I have to make this work. I have one goal in mind and I cannot cock it up. I want a prescription for risperidone. How do I know about this antipsychotic drug that is rarely used on children? Because unbeknownst to you, you have a guardian angel here on earth. She's a cousin and a doctor and a beautiful human being and I have been feeding her information about your symptoms over the phone without you knowing. She went to talk to colleagues in the mental health field and then gave me the intel I needed. When I have told Dr V everything about the voices, hallucinations, paranoia, sleeplessness and terror, I come and get you. She examines you so gently, so kindly and so beautifully reassuringly, without firing a single uncomfortable question your way. Then she tells you to go back out, and rapidly gives me her medical diagnosis.

"She needs risperidone," says Dr V. I want to do a victory dance; this is the moment we've been waiting for. "But," she warns me, "I can't prescribe it." I deflate.

"I will put in an acute referral to see a psychiatrist and have an appointment for her by the end of day."

So close. We hobble out on to a busy London road.

London is an assault to the senses at the best of times. Through the eyes and ears of a psychotic child, it is a protracted, violent, bloody one. The sirens are constant. You are agitated and frightened by the sound. An ambulance speeds past us. You stop.

"Someone is having a really bad day," you say, staring after it. Bereft. Paralyzed.

"Or a good one," I reply, "those sirens mean help is on hand." You look at me with such a faraway, lost expression.

"But they're driving away from the hospital."

This is so classic you. Ever the sentinel, clocking danger, noticing everything. The bad sticking like Velcro. The good slipping off as if you were made of Teflon.

The pavements are thick with Christmas shoppers. Bikes swerve in and out of traffic, making you swerve in unison. Buses bear down on us, looming as huge as they did when you were a newborn baby, perilously close. I've pounded these pavements my whole life, and I have never felt scared in this magnificent city. I pray it won't betray me now. We take the back streets, keep to the tree-lined residential areas and zigzag our way back to the office that we've temporarily set up home in. I've just got to keep you calm till the afternoon, then I can hand over that responsibility to the magic of medicine.

We are watching *Glee* when Dr V calls me. She's apologetic. She's going to try another avenue tomorrow.

You look at me with great suspicion.

The following day, Dr V calls back.

"I am so sorry," she says, "there isn't one child psychiatrist with a free two-hour appointment, which is what is required."

You are looking at me. Beady-eyed.

"Watch *Glee*," I say, and step on to the fire escape.

"The child psychiatrist I wanted you to see isn't available until mid-January," says Dr V.

Nausea swells up. I am operating from one hour to the next. The fifteenth of January may as well be in another millennium. To get help, you have to get in line, and at Christmas, it's a long line.

"What am I going to do? I've promised her she'll get help."

"I think you should go to A&E," says Dr V.

We're back to A&E? What if they sectioned you and you were placed miles away? I can't do that to you after everything that has happened. I am thinking fast, breathing faster and I can feel myself shaking. I look at you, bundled up under a furry blanket, holding a furry pillow, cocooned as safely as I can cocoon you in this brash, noisy city. But you are not watching *Glee*. You are watching me. I smile back at you, put on a reassuring sing-song voice, and Dr V and I come up with a plan.

I go back in and tell you the news.

"Let's go," you say. "I can go to A&E. I think we should go."

I talk you out of it. I will never know what that decision cost you.

My mother comes to do a puzzle with you so I can go to a cafe and put the plan into action without your paranoid ears trained on my every word. I make a begging call to the medical secretary of the psychiatrist Dr V recommends. I send her an email explaining our situation and beg to be put on a cancellation list. I speak to the lead psychiatrist of CAMHS at Chelsea and Westminster Hospital and assure her that I will take you to A&E should your condition deteriorate. I order a second cup of coffee, which I shouldn't drink, as I am jacked up on enough adrenaline and cortisol to run a marathon, but I want to extend this unguarded moment alone. Slowly, I walk back, hug my mother and continue to eke out the minutes watching *Glee*, doing puzzles and waiting till I can slip you the strongest dose of lorazepam allowed, hold your hand in the dark and recite my favourite poem to you over and over until you slide into a comatose sleep.

WHAH, WHAH, WHAH.

We both leap up, throw the duvet off and run ... to where?

WHAH, WHAH, WHAH.

The fire alarm in the building is deafening. You are instantly terrified. Finally, it is happening – you are going to burn alive. We put our shoes on, I grab keys, open the door, smell for smoke.

"It is probably a false alarm," I say. I am thinking, *It would be just my luck if it wasn't.*

WHAH, WHAH, WHAH.

You're crying. I've got to get you out. I take your hand.

"Stay with me, I'll keep you safe." These promises I keep making that I have no right to make.

We are halfway down the stairs—

WHAH, WHAH. It stops. We stop.

It probably only lasted a few minutes, but the impact is huge.

"We're not safe," you say. "We're not safe," your eyes darting manically.

"Let's go back in," I say.

You look at me. "It's not safe here. Why did you take me out of the hospital? Why didn't you leave me there? What's wrong with you?"

You are spiralling and fast. Your head is flicking this way and that, listening to warnings I cannot hear.

"We need to leave now!"

I consider this. We could go to a hotel, we could go for a walk, but it's the middle of the night, we're at the end of a long dark cul-de-sac, and this part of London isn't all leafy avenues and well-lit houses. It's shady. That's why I like it. Normally.

"What if there is a fire?" There is a long list of what ifs.

"I'll go and check," I say.

"Don't leave me …" You grab me hard. You are wild-eyed. You are not you. I am losing; the people are winning. It dawns on me where we must go. Gently, I try to take your hand.

"Roxy, honey, I think we should go to A&E."

"NOOOOOOO." Every reason I had ever given you was repeated back to me, with a touch of venom and a coating of mistrust:

"You said they might send me away."

"You said they'll put me on an adult ward."

"You said you might not be able to stay."

I cannot take you to A&E because I cannot get you there. You pull away and retreat to a dark corner. A watchful, wounded beast, tuned in to a psychotic radio wave, warning of danger. Your eyes narrow when I approach. I am the danger.

I should have taken you in when I had the chance. I said I could keep you safe. It was a lie.

THE NOISE AND HASTE

My granny comes to see me and we do a puzzle. I even buy a puzzle with XL pieces so that she can see them properly. Then I watch more *Glee*.

I wish that I could tell you more. I want to describe to you what psychosis feels like. There are so many gaps. Whole days have just vanished. Sometimes it is more specific than that, hours and minutes have vanished. It is terrifying, really. The actual feeling of knowing that something has happened but not being able to visualize it. I trust that you are telling the truth, but you could just as easily not be. I wouldn't know. I don't understand how I can remember specific details like what I had for breakfast, but then I have no recollection of going into CAMHS and lying in the foetal position on the floor.

There are voices, and sometimes it is a voice inside of me, it is coming from my head and it tells me that I need to do things. That isn't a new voice, though. I have always had that voice telling me that I am not safe at night, telling me to sleep with hockey sticks, telling me that if I don't turn off my iPod at an exact time on an exact song, something bad will happen. So that voice has always been with me, but that voice is different now, it is more overwhelming. Before, that voice was anxiety – and I think I knew that. Of course, it terrified me and I still had to do what it said, but I knew that it was anxiety. Now, I can't stand up to that voice. That voice is completely overwhelming me. That voice inside my head dictates what I need to do and if I don't do it, then ... well, not doing it just isn't an option. That voice doesn't feel like a part of me any more. That voice has gotten inside of me and it is stuck there and I feel like a puppet and it is a puppet master moving my arms around and opening my mouth. Before, I felt like it was me against my own brain, but this isn't my brain, this is something darker and more evil and it is inside me. It is impossible to explain, which is why I am rambling on like a crazy person. Then there are these other voices which come from outside. They tell me what to do.

Like trains, for example. Trains. What is it about trains? I have never particularly liked trains, I never had a toy train or a train set when I was younger, but the street we used to live on ran along a train line and the house shook a bit as they rumbled past at night. They are just moving vehicles that I use to get from one place to another and now I am told that I have to go to them. I have to sit at the barriers and I watch the trains, and every time a train leaves it is a personal attack – they are leaving me. I feel so alone when that train pulls out of the station. There is always stomping and banging and feet in the flat above us in the night. Outside our window is a train track and I hear the trains go past as they leave me, and the whole ground shakes. And they are shaking me and they are leaving me and the people upstairs are jumping up and down and up and down because they want to scare me. They do scare me. These people don't want me to sleep. Sleep is not safe. You want me to sleep. The people manage to snake their way into my sleep, my dreams. My sleep is not quiet and peaceful, it is noisy and chaotic. I am still shouted at, still teased. Sleep is not a safe place for me, it is this great unknown where I have no protection from the overwhelming voices. You give me pills and try to coax me into sleep. You recite "Desiderata" to me over and over again. It is beautiful. I focus on memorizing each line slowly and carefully. The words of the poem break through the barrier of jumbled voices. Eventually, I start to drift off and I pray that I will enter a world of quiet.

"Remember what peace there may be in silence."

I really need some silence.

CHRISTMAS ANGELS

The NSPCC Christmas angels are hung the length of Regent Street and Oxford Street and you are bedazzled by them. So much so, you want to stay and talk to them. You stare up at them, the sparkling white lights reflected in your eyes. You look happy.

I am happy to let you because I've left plenty of time to make the appointment. I think I'm covered for all eventualities, though I didn't have talking angels on my list.

"They are so beautiful," you say, mesmerized.

I check my watch. Five more minutes, then we have to go. It has been like this for days. We have navigated our way around London as I have narrated in your ear what is happening. I make split-second decisions constantly, weighing up options. Crossing a busy London road with a shuffling child is difficult, even when the green man says go. Especially when The People say no.

"I want to stay and talk to my friends," you say.

I move the chess pieces around in my head. We can't miss this appointment. It's everything I've been working towards. Dr B: child and adolescent psychiatrist.

"We'll come back," I say, facing upwards. "We'll see your friends later." I put my arm through yours. "You are right, they are very beautiful."

I've been communicating directly with The People for a while now, why not angels too? We shuffle along the pavement.

This is the assessment we've been waiting for. I need you to answer all the questions, however hard.

It's risky to mention questions. You hate questions. You start to slow up. I've pushed too hard. No doubt The People are telling you not to go – they are walking towards their own demise.

"I want to go back to the angels," you plead.

I put my arm around you and push you onwards.

"Later," I say, "we'll go back later."

"Promise?"

"I promise."

Exactly one month since you were sent home from school with the instruction not to leave you alone, and one week since we took you out of a psychiatric unit, we walk into Dr B's plush office. We have, in that month, not let you be alone. You are sick of me. The two-hour assessment is horrendous. You try your best to answer his questions, but you appear not to really understand. You glare at Dr B as if he is the enemy or stupid, or both. I suspect The People are drowning him out, but you are afraid to mention them. Perhaps they have told you something terrible will happen if you snitch on them. I have to fill in the blanks even though I had emailed every sordid detail to him. Hearing me tell your story makes you hate me all over again, especially since there are still things that I didn't know until reading this book. You don't put me right, you just despise me for being wrong. I believe you think I am betraying you, but all I am trying to do is leave with what we came for and if that means you hating me, then that is a price I am willing to pay. Parenting isn't a popularity contest.

There have been so many false finishing lines and this is just another one. "The end is where we start from," wrote Kurt Vonnegut, and he was right. We end this miserable period of illness and begin a miserable period of recovery which looks very similar to illness.

He tells you to wait downstairs.

"So?" I ask expectantly. "What's going on?"

"It is clear she is experiencing some form of psychosis, there is clear detachment, paranoia, and she is presenting as disso-ciative. But –"

No, no, no buts, just give us the drugs…

"I don't like giving medical diagnoses because children's brains are so fluid and they change. This is good, because it means they can make full recoveries. It is important not to label her as anything – sometimes labels mean children get stuck. Mental illnesses begin small and grow without treatment, you don't wake up one morning schizophrenic …"

He goes on talking. This is all really key, I realize only later, but at the time, all I want to know is: Have you passed the assessment? Do we get antipsychotic drugs or do I go on feeding you an assorted version of benzodiazepines?

You pass. All he had to do was look you in the eye and he could see that you were a malfunctioning human. Your irises are pinpricks, even in the subdued lighting of the psychiatrist's office. The light isn't penetrating your soul. You are engulfed in darkness. I walk out victorious: on stiff cream paper, headed with the name of a man with more letters than the alphabet after it, is a flurry of ink from a weighty pen. The magic word for the magic pill: risperidone. Halle-fucking-lujah.

You are exhausted after the meeting and swallowed again by sadness as we shuffle to the pharmacy two blocks down the road. We've come so far, but I swear getting you down these two blocks nearly breaks me.

There is a circular burgundy faux-leather seat. You lie across it, defeated. Whatever was left in you, it's gone, leaving the carcass of the girl my daughter once was wrapped in a thick black puffa jacket. I go to the counter and wait for the packet of pills. The pharmacist is a kind man who doesn't mind you are draped over his furniture.

"Very good medication," he says. Kindness feeds me.

I open the packet, split the foil, crack the magic bean in half and, with a peach tea from the drinks fridge, give you the first dose. Then we hail a cab and get you home. Another promise broken. You'd never make it back to the angels.

While you watch *Glee*, I watch you for signs. As long as there are no immediate side effects, I can give you a second, stronger dose that night. I read the small print. The possible side effects range from Parkinson's disease through to coma due to uncommon diabetes.

Jeez, this better work.

At 9 p.m., having watched you like a hawk, I feel confident enough to give you the second dose. One whole magic bean plus two melatonin. Dr B has explained to us both that in order to heal, your brain must be put into a deep sleep, the sort of sleep you probably haven't had for months, probably years, possibly ever. The goal is to up the dose until you are sleeping for 12 to 13 hours a night. You take the pill and get into bed. You are a 14-year-old girl in pyjamas and a Pooh Bear dressing gown and my heart breaks for you because Dr B has told me that he estimates recovery will take six months.

It takes over a year.

*

Men push wheelbarrows out of a first-floor window and pour rubble into a skip on the pavement. Bricks bounce off the metal interior of the skip and echo loudly. Radio 2 blasts out of a Black+Decker radio. The banter is louder still. Your sleep is closing in on a miraculous 10 hours a night and you seem stronger physically, but mentally you are still vulnerable. I don't think walking under scaffolding rumbling with noise and crawling with builders is a good idea. I lead you on to the road, it's a cul-de-sac, so I don't think you'll feel threatened. A car is idling at the top. Idling. The driver appears to be staring at us as we walk up the road. I don't like the look in his eyes. Suddenly, he is revving his engine. I dismiss the threat – it's a cul-de-sac, he can't go anywhere. We are halfway past the skip when the driver, this stranger, suddenly accelerates and swerves towards us. You run. I am apoplectic with rage, and when he turns around and drives back, I photograph his numberplate. He shouts something sexist and threatening to me and I shout back that I am taking his details to the police. It feels good to rage, shout, make a noise, stand up for myself. I look around. You've gone. How could I have been so stupid and reckless? I scan the street. It takes me a few terrifying seconds to locate you. You are cowering alone behind a car. Your eyes roll in terror. I gather you back up, but you're cross and pull away.

"That was so stupid, why did you do that?!"

"Sorry, honey, I'm sorry."

"That woman thinks you're mad!"

"What woman?" I ask.

There's the look again. I am the danger. You don't trust me to keep you safe and despite all the hours of gentle care, I keep slipping up and in doing so, prove you right.

It is only the lure of the NSPCC Christmas angels that gets you back to Dr B. He needs to see the effects of the medication. Although you've begged for treatment, you dread the appointments and actively dislike him. I go in alone first to fill him in and then I sit with you when he talks to you. You want me there for now. You don't trust me, but you trust him less. You are reticent and tight-lipped; I watch as he tries to draw blood from the hunched stone on his sofa. If it wasn't so prohibitively expensive and we weren't so desperate, it would be almost funny watching a reputable, highly trained psychiatrist try to crack you. But it's not funny, it's annoying. Sometimes, just sometimes, I wonder if maybe you have nothing to say.

We are back on Regent Street, a Starbucks warming our hands.

"Dr B can't help you if you don't tell him what is going on," I snap.

We are seeing your friends in daylight for the first time.

"They're cross," you say.

"No, they're not." I kick myself. "I mean, how do you know they're cross?"

"They aren't being very nice," you say.

I look at them. With their frames visible, the angels look more skeletal. I can see why you are frightened.

"They are saying mean things."

Where have I heard that before? *Mummy, there are horrible rumours going around about me at school ...*

They were calling you names then, and they are calling you names now. Your friends have turned against you, angels no longer.

Dr B's written assessment arrives in the post. He admits it is hard to comprehensively diagnose while you are this unresponsive, but he offers his opinion.

Roxy's hallucinatory symptoms could be interpreted as an equivalent of her emotional experience of being in the school environment knowing that her peers have viewed intimate pictures of her. As Roxy put it, these peers were hostile in their language towards her. The hallucinations she reports are "people" with hurtful intentions.

Your friends called you names, others shouted insults without showing their faces. The People and now the angels have followed you out of your real life and are crucifying you with dark imaginings. They haunt you and taunt you – but they aren't the only dark angel.

The letter continues:

Alongside these events in school, her behaviour became very defiant and challenging at home and until the month of November were met by angry reactions from her parents who were very unaware of what was going on. This no doubt led Roxy to feel isolated with her family equally.

Every year when those NSPCC angels go up, you and I can barely look at them. All I see are rows of beautiful demons, like the angel of death at the end of *Raiders of the Lost Ark*, bearing down, sucking your soul. I also see me – at my impatient, frustrated, exhausted worst.

ANGELS AND DEMONS

The angels are talking to me, but I can't see their mouths moving. Their mouths aren't moving, but these sounds are coming out of them. Sometimes they are nice and sometimes they are mean. I know they are mean. I can sense things watching me and following me and I can sense this danger and I know that people are being mean. I can hear what they are saying, but it's not really like they are saying them. I know it is the angels. That doesn't make much sense. Their voices are different, they are lighter and colder and meaner, they have this tang. Sometimes they are my friends and sometimes they turn against me. The angels don't even look like angels. They are more like golden Dementors stretching up above me. Watching. I don't think that they are real angels, if angels even can be real, they are lights made out of electricity and metal and plastic. I know that. They still say such personal things to me, these pieces of metal. They tell me to slow down and to not go to the psychiatrist. He will judge me for all the bad things I did.

You tell the doctor about the photos and the running away and the social services and the self-harm and the people. I sound like such an awful person when you say it all together. I don't make eye contact with the doctor. I cannot explain the photos or the running away or the self-harm or the people. I can't explain any of it to him, so I just don't speak. I can't explain how I'm feeling.

I leave the room so that you can talk to him and I go to the bathroom. I do not like going to the toilet. I don't like going to any bathrooms really. Why do all the bathrooms have mirrors? Why do you need a mirror to wash your hands and go to the loo? Why were mirrors even invented? I do not need to look at myself when I wash my hands. I don't want to look myself in the eye, so I stare down at the water pouring over my hands. The soap stings because I have so many little cuts around my fingernails. I don't dare look up. I don't want to see all that stuff that everybody has seen. So I look down and I scrub my hands and I bite my lip through the sharp sting of the soap. I turn around, still looking at the floor as I walk out. I shut the door on that awful reflection. When I am older, I'm not going to have any mirrors in my house.

MEDS ARE GOOD, BUT THERE AIN'T NO MAGIC PILL

The People stay for Christmas. I invite them in and then tiptoe around them like a grumpy uncle asleep in the corner. Do not wake the beast. The meds seep into your system slowly. We have to build up the quantity milligram by milligram; it's not yet enough to extinguish the voices. During the day, you exist upstairs in my bedroom. We create a sanctuary for you with a TV and puzzles, food on a tray, music and books. We have two goals: keeping you calm and building up your sleep. We need you sleeping at least 12 hours a night. You're managing about nine. It's not enough. Like an ill person, you have occasional quiet, solo visitors. Unlike an ill person, your illness is never openly discussed.

Downstairs, Christmas lunch is laid for two aunts, two uncles, five cousins, three grannies, two grandfathers, two sisters and two parents. There is a flurry of activity coming from the kitchen, my mother's carrots versus my sister's mother-in-law's potatoes, popping corks, loud, overexcited children, crackers. Last Christmas was wrapped in tragedy. They want this Christmas to be fun. This is one of the hardest days of your illness. No wonder it is statistically the busiest day of the year for heart surgeons. My heart is creaking under the strain of holding in your sorrow and pouring forth joy for your sisters. It's the contrast that kills. I hear a little voice ...

"Mummy ..."

You don't like being on your own for very long.

I go back up to sit with you in bed and pretend a party isn't going on downstairs without you. Downstairs, your dad does the same in reverse and then we swap over. Everyone pretends there isn't an ill child hearing voices lying broken upstairs, but we can hear your quiet wailing and occasional shouts whenever there is a lull in the conversation. It's miserable, and though I join the lunch, my heart isn't really in it; the turkey sticks in my throat. So I re-enter the cocoon we've created – there isn't really room for anyone else inside it, and outside it I feel as flimsy as a butterfly's wing.

"I want to go back to London. I can't do this. It's too noisy," you say.

You are getting angry that I can come and go and you cannot. You think I am so lucky. I don't feel very lucky. I try to tell you that people are capable of overcoming atrocity and adversity and I believe you will get through this.

"You don't know what you're talking about, your life is perfect."

I am trying to be helpful. I am trying to give you perspective. I tell you I was raped by my first boyfriend. I was 16 and it messed with my head because I continued to go out with him and told myself it hadn't happened. I know shame and self-loathing. You will recover. It is a horrible conversation and completely backfires.

You start asking me when actual treatment will start. Fair enough, I took you out of a treatment centre. For what? For nothing? I try to explain that treatment doesn't start until the meds work. We are in another holding pattern and – have I mentioned? – it's Christmas. Even psychiatrists get time off. Instead, we separate you from the group, away from the noise and the triggers. Away from the fun. You are increasingly agitated.

"Why do you keep moving the furniture?"

No one is moving furniture, I think. "Probably just the wind," I say.

"Mama?"

I look up from my computer.

"Who are you talking to?"

I haven't been talking to anyone. The house is empty.

"Mama, who's shouting?"

No one is shouting. And what's with this "Mama" thing?

Those 10 days in London limping towards the appointment were hard, the 12 days of Christmas waiting for the meds to work are harder still. Your hope is crushed. I first notice the change in your voice pattern at bedtime. You start to sound like a child. You then start to act like a child. You want to sit on my knee.

"Oh, Mama," says the odd, spooky doll, cutting off my blood circulation.

This freaks me out, so I call Dr B. We head to London for an appointment. You are reticent with him, suspicious as always. I find I gain more intelligence when you leave the room.

"The little-girl voice is a form of regression," he explains. "A common symptom of a breakdown. She has regressed to where she was when felt safest."

"Four years old?" I ask.

"What happened when she was four?"

The memory is sudden and vivid. I am having contractions, so I ask our part-time nanny to collect you from nursery. I hear you both come into the flat, but you don't bound into the sitting room where I am timing the early seismic tremors. Finally, I go in search of you. She has you in the steamy shower room. You can't breathe.

"It's her chest," says the nanny. She is very young. Experienced, yes, but a child in charge of a child. "Croup, maybe?"

Your breathing is getting more and more laboured. I swear your lips are going blue. I make a rough calculation; we jump in the car and still in my dressing gown, I drive 10 minutes to A&E. I carry you in. You've passed out by this time. Within seconds, they have you on oxygen and steroids and in 20 minutes, you are fine again.

"It isn't croup," says the nurse. "More like a panic attack. Anything scare her?"

That's when I realize my contractions have stopped dead. I will never know what the nanny said to you on the way home, but whatever it was, it terrified you.

Before siblings, you were the epicentre of our universe, and your every need was met. By the time you turned five, you had two new sisters, a new school, a new house and a nanny you did not like. So yes, that's what happened when you were four.

"An essential part of growing up is learning to meet your own needs and regulate your own emotions," he says. "She's going to have to learn to do that for herself. It isn't going to be easy."

"When do you think she'll be able to go back to school?"

He looks at me forlornly. I clearly haven't understood. He explains again what has happened to your brain. He explains again how long it will take to heal. He tells me sleep is key.

"I don't think she'll make it back this academic year," he says.

I take my teenage four-year-old home, dose her up and wait for sleep to soothe her misfiring brain. I lie beside you. I recite my poem. Sleep, my baby, sleep.

"Sleep."

"I can't sleep."

Sometimes I give you melatonin, on top of lorazepam, on top of risperidone. It's a sledgehammer, I know, but I just need you to sleep.

"I'm having bad dreams."

This is true. You thrash and yelp, tremor and whimper. Sometimes a hand on your back is enough to calm you. Sometimes you wake, scared and lost, sometimes suspicious and cross, some-times meek and mild and we pad downstairs, make hot milk, then begin the process again. Your mood flips and all I can do is hold your hand, recite my poem. "Go placidly," I begin, and try to lead you across the boundary of consciousness to where your brain can heal.

"Sleep."

The irony of ironies: that dark quiet place you have feared for so long is in fact where you'll find salvation.

CHRISTMAS

There are so many excited kids screaming and running around. It is too much noise and too much movement for me. Then I am angry with myself because I cannot ruin this happy day for them, for my sisters particularly. I grit my teeth and I beg the voices to stop. I try desperately to focus on the person in front of me but I cannot listen to the words they are saying. Covering my ears doesn't help; these voices aren't coming in through my ears.

I am in my parents' bedroom trying to distract myself. Christmas is going on downstairs without me. I don't like being up here by myself. I make a collage and try to focus on the television. It isn't working, so I lie in bed and try to sit with these voices. Sometimes I get so cross with them that I can't help but shout, "GO AWAY!". When you are gone, I want you here, but when you are with me, I feel angry that you can't fix this and guilty that I am keeping you from the party.

I come join everyone for a little bit, but I can't focus on anybody speaking to me. My granny tries to ask me questions and have a conversation with me and I so want to be normal, but I cannot do it. I feel like there are hundreds of speakers around my head all blasting different things, and I can't decipher any of them, it is just an army of overwhelming sound. I open my new shoes and go back upstairs.

I am cross with you. I hate that you would rather be downstairs than with me even though I know that makes perfect sense. I want to shout at you and hit you.

Why do the voices always shout at me? Why don't they shout at you?

You are so lucky that you get to smile and sing and eat with everybody.

It is so unfair and you are so lucky.

You shout back.

"Roxy. You have no idea what you're talking about. Everything wasn't perfect and happy for me. I was raped when I was 16."

You shout back and then you leave. We don't speak about it again.

I am in bed by 6 p.m., like a baby. I don't like Christmas.

We are having Boxing Day dinner at my granny's house. I put on my nice clothes and I try to act normal. I sit there and I pretend that it is quiet in my head and I try to listen. I go outside to breathe and when I come back in, my cousin is stuffing something under the table. She is trying to hide it from me. It is a family necklace that my granny has given her. My granny doesn't give me a necklace. She doesn't like me any more.

KILLER COCKTAIL

On a blisteringly cold morning in January 2017, we drop your sisters off at school and take ourselves to a cafe. From now on, your life will be lived without you. Instead, you will be here, with me, wherever I am, stuck.

"When will I be able to go back to school?" you ask in your little girl voice.

I duck the question and order coffee for me, tea for you. I look at my watch. It isn't even 9 a.m. Already I can feel the drag

on time. How can I tell you this may go on for months? A year?
I can't compute it myself.

Two women congregate at the counter wearing Lycra, waiting
to be seated. One of them is Ryan the maths geek's mother. You
look terror-stricken and shrink in the chair. I force myself to
witter on inanely. I smile at you. I do not make eye contact
with them, nor do they with me. I feel like a specimen in a
tank. Visible, but separated. Does anyone even know how shit
this all is? For both of us. I know where they are going: to an
exercise class I used to bounce off to myself. Now I live off
caffeine, alcohol and adrenaline. It's a killer cocktail.

As the women walk past our table, I notice you are digging
your single remaining thumb nail into the back of your
hand, you've gnawed the rest off. The soft pale pink skin is
pocked with dark red crescent-moon cut-outs; your own cookie
cutter of pain, etching out your days in solitude. I want to slap
your hand away so much that I sit on my own and try not to
look sad. This is going to be our greatest challenge. We can't
stay in our kitchen with the dog, puzzles and the Aga all day,
but evidence of your former life is wallpapered on to every part
of this town, and seeing it sends you into a tailspin, followed
by a crash. You are left in pieces. My job is to weld the pieces
back together. It is painful; I cause you pain. But what choice
do I have? You must, you must trudge on. I pay and we get up
to go for a walk. I see another mother walking towards us and
instinctively lower my head. I needn't have bothered. She took
one look at us and scurried across the road.

Our early-morning saviour is wearing brown suede moccasins.
I can tell he has ended up walking by accident – he is walking with
us so we don't have to walk alone. Who else would walk in moccasins in January? He slips and slides in the mud, reminding me of

a Quentin Blake illustration of Tom beating Captain Najork. He is a sensitive soul who has been through his own difficulties and luckily for us, is there to catch us when we land in a lump at his feet. For six months, you steal his breakfast and for six months, he lets you and over that time we become firm friends. We love him. And his dog – mustn't forget Bolt, even if he does pee in the corner of the cafe. These are precious moments, flashes of light in the dark night that are now our days. I hang on to these moments with gratitude and hope, but the truth is no matter how many almond milk lattes I drink and how many blueberry muffins you steal, we are largely left to our own devices, limping to the next appointment with the psychiatrist, crawling through time.

"She has started producing breast milk," I say quietly, though I have left you in the waiting room. You do not want to be present for this conversation. It is too embarrassing. I've washed the concentric rings off the inside of your bras, but it keeps coming. It really upsets you.

"Imagine how the boys feel," Dr B replies.

I shake my head; I don't understand. He explains.

"Risperidone causes the pituitary gland to produce excessive prolactin, the hormone that promotes breast growth and milk production. It's actually more common in boys because they are prescribed risperidone more often than girls."

"Why?"

"When boys become unwell, they are more likely to become dysregulated and pose more of a threat to others."

You are just a risk to yourself, I think. We've made a deal with the devil. Voices for breast milk.

"So what next? We can't just go on like this."

Actually, that is exactly what we must do. We must limp on, like this, week after week, month after month. Recovery is glacial and to be honest, at this point, it hasn't even started. You are still acute. I just don't know it. Dr B keeps trying to tell me, but I can't compute.

I call you into the appointment and you take your place, your back squeezed into the corner of the sofa and stare at him through your narrowed eyelids – all suspicion and coiled loathing. He explains the hormone imbalance. You're not impressed. I actually start to feel a bit sorry for the man. A million hours of study, for this?

"I would like you to see a neurosurgeon," he says.

Your eyes widen. You sit up a fraction straighter. I know what you're thinking: maybe there is another explanation for what has happened to you. What a crazy world we are in, where a brain tumour has an upside – but I understand it, too. Mental illness is nebulous, ethereal and hard to pin down. It's a feeling that can't be felt by any other. There isn't an operation or a bone to fix, and visitors don't bring chocolates and flowers. But a brain tumour – well, that would explain everything. That would mean you can hold your head up high. Suddenly, you like Dr B. It doesn't last.

MILK AND SUGAR

One foot in front of the other. Don't trip. Don't trip. I just need to make it to the cafe.

We are only one street away from the cafe. One single street that seems to be getting longer and longer with every second. This town knows me. The buildings and the people know me. I stare at the pavement and focus on avoiding the cracks. If I don't make eye contact with the people around me, then they don't exist. I need to see how far the cafe is. Surely we are close now.

Just one look, Roxy.

I hold my breath and glance up at the street in front of me just in time to make eye contact with a woman I know. She promptly looks away and crosses to the other side of the road. It isn't even subtle.

Do not cry, Roxy. Do not cry.

I am practically hanging off you now.

I am so dirty and disgusting that people cross the street. They cross the street to avoid the mental slut who broke, as if this may be catching.

I go back to tracing the cracks on the pavement and I imagine myself building a dam across my tear ducts. I force the salty water back into my soul.

I feel worse now that the medication has started to work. I am being brought back to reality and I hate reality. It is just me and you and my thoughts. With the people gone, there is no distraction.

Finally, I collapse in the armchair in the corner of the cafe. It is 8.30 a.m. and I am exhausted. I gather all my remaining energy and pull my eyes up from my lap. I look around the cafe. No children, obviously – everybody is at school. The head of pastoral care's husband. Aiden's aunt. Ryan's mum. These faces make the room spin and my heart race and I start to sweat.

I dig at the hole I've created in my hand. Scooping out crescent-shaped slices of skin.

I pull at my earring, imagining the beautiful pain if it ripped through my lobe.

"Roxy, what do you want? Tea? Coffee?"

I can't speak. I especially can't shout my order to you across this room of piranhas. I manage only a small shake of my head. You order your first almond milk latte.

My leg shakes, my hand shakes. I keep building that dam to stop the tears. You sit down across from me and try to pretend that I'm not cracking in the seat next to you. Maybe if you don't acknowledge it, then it isn't happening.

"I know you said that you didn't want anything, but sometimes we just need a cup of tea with sugar."

Charlotte places a mug, a gingerbread man and a small pot of sugar cubes in front of me. She works here every morning. She must know something is wrong because I'm not at school and I look like a china doll, but she speaks to me like a normal teenager. Not like I'm sick. Charlotte, thank you.

The sugary tea works, my leg stops moving and I stop attacking my own body. I begin to breathe.

These people are not thinking about you. They are thinking about their own lives and their own family and their own problems. It is in your head, Roxy.

Bolt pushes open the door and comes charging into the cafe dragging his besotted owner. He sniffs around the customers, collects his treat from Charlotte, lifts his leg to pee on the spider plant in the corner and then tries to kiss me all over my face. Then his owner comes in and kisses me on the cheek.

"Good morning, darlings."

He runs us through his latest ailment and work problem and then Charlotte brings his usual.

A blueberry muffin.

He eats half, I steal the other half. Every single morning.

He talks and talks and I actually laugh. I feel normal.

The tea has rushed to my bladder and now I desperately need to pee. The bathroom is on the other side of the cafe, and to reach it I have to walk through the narrow space between the tables of chattering parents with judgemental eyes and slicing whispers. I jiggle around in my seat, holding it in for a while until the discomfort turns into stomach pain.

I take a deep breath and stand up. I look at the floor and start to walk down the room. Immediately, I am back at school, walking through the shouts and the whispers and the looks. I bow my head lower.

Nobody is thinking about you, Roxy.

I am now so stooped that I am practically crawling. They are not thinking about you. Don't trip. Nobody says anything to me but they might as well be throwing rotten tomatoes and booing. That is what is happening in my head.

I make it to the bathroom and thank my legs for not letting me fall. I made it. I look at myself in the mirror, which is something I rarely do nowadays. My lips are scabbed over and there is dried blood around them. There are white flecks all over my hair and scalp. I look like I have walked through a snow machine. It doesn't seem to matter how often I scrub my scalp with Head & Shoulders, the dandruff keeps coming. It's the medication.

You order coffee after coffee after coffee, anything to delay having to go home. You look longingly at the people who walk past, silently begging people to invite us on a walk, or to have another coffee – anything.

When the cafe is empty and the lunch menus have been put out, we eventually have to go back to our kitchen. There is one large window which looks out on to a field and under the window-sill is a ripped floral two-seater sofa. Your desk and the kitchen table are next to the sofa and the floor in this part of the room is wooden. The other half has a kitchen island and an Aga. The Aga is the only heat, so I spend a lot of time sat on the dog bed next to it. It is a big room but, Jesus, it feels so, so small. The most I do is move between the sofa, the dog bed, the fridge, and the kitchen table. I try to move to a different spot every couple of hours so it doesn't get too repetitive. The other rooms are too cold to spend time in.

I try to do some of the geography worksheets sent by the school. I can't do them and then I get angry and then sad. I teach myself a new chord on the guitar and try to play the three songs that I know. My hands shake a lot, so I struggle to keep my fingers pressed down on the strings.

I tell you that I have a headache and then add the paracetamol to the little pot in my bedside table. I'm never going to take these pills, of course; it just comforts me to know that they are there.

I spend some time on the collage I've been making. I stick magazine cut-outs on to cardboard and then connect them with unfolded paper clips.

I take off my bra to get into my pyjamas. There are dark patches on the inside. My boobs are wet. Shit.

My weird triangular boobs are leaking. Milk.

I hate this medication.

SNOW GLOBE

The fabulously eccentric neurosurgeon assesses you in a nano-second and dismisses your need for a brain scan with the flick of her hand.

"Boys are bastards, girls are bitches – do not let them steal one more day," she tells you. "They are not worth it."

Just like that, our drama is reduced to nothing with an expressive Latin shrug. Everything else has been a storm in a snow globe. In the two hours you talk to this lady, the snow settles. You can see the landscape of your life clearly for the first time in six months. Nothing is as bad as it seems. We walk out pretty chipper, even though you don't have a brain tumour.

Instead, you are started on a course of non-invasive brain surgery. With the help of a London-based dialectical behaviour therapist attached to Dr B's clinic. You will learn to rewire your brain using a combination of behavioural therapies that are designed to give the patient skills to deal with their extreme and acute emotions. The trouble is this cure means constantly shaking the snow globe, which leaves you standing alone locked inside a frozen storm that's raging all over again. It's one step forward, three steps back. There are only two places for that rage to go. It's you or me. At first, the rage is mostly directed at yourself. Watching you attack your own body makes me want to shake you. Don't you know how precious you are, how beautiful you are, how miraculous your body is? You are sad all the time and you have a lot of time to be sad.

"Remember what the neurologist said: Don't let them steal one more minute, let alone a day."

You glare at me. *What the fuck do you know?* You don't have to say it. I know what you are thinking.

A million times a day, I feel I am pulling your hand away from a bloody spot.

"Stop!" you snap.

You stop! I want to shout back childishly.

Pick, pick, pick. I have to look away, it makes you look so – I can barely think it – damaged.

You peel strips of translucent skin off your bee-stung lips. You dig out skin on the palms of your hands. You pick the same patch of scalp on your head until it bleeds. It is not a spectator sport, yet I have no choice but to watch. We remain glued at the hip. I find it almost impossible to say nothing.

Of course I say something.

"Flick the elastic band instead," I venture.

It is the wrong thing.

Your rage relocates, locked once again on me. "You know nothing."

Another time, it's: "What's wrong with you?"

Sometimes, I get: "You don't understand!"

Followed by: "You don't even try to understand!"

And finally: "You have no heart."

"What's wrong with you?" I hear that one a lot. For months. Other times, it is just steely silence. You look daggers at me. I can feel them bore through my back as I sit at my desk, just a few feet from the two-seater sofa that you and the dog occupy for hours every day. I know what you are thinking: *It's alright for you, you have a life, I have nothing.* But my life is your life. Even when I am at script meetings, I am thinking about you. When I copy-edit a project, I am thinking about you. Always, always trying to find that missing piece of the puzzle, trying to stay one step ahead of your kaleidoscopic mind, trying to hold you up until you are strong enough to hold yourself.

You collapse on to the floor, the dog curls herself inside the curve of your body, places a paw on your arm and stares into your eyes. Thank God for the dog. I call the dialectical behaviour therapist in London. Throughout your recovery, I have found a backchannel to her. She tells me nothing, of course – client confidentiality – but I need her to know what is going on our end because without a full diagnosis, we are still trying to piece this all together. I tell her everything.

"What do I do? I don't know what to do."

"Just make sure she knows you are there for her, no matter what."

I crouch down and touch your shoulder. You turn your head and look up at me.

"I need your strong," you say, sounding lost and far away.

You do need my strong, and I need my strong. I took you out of the psychiatric unit. I decided to take on the role of guard, nurse, therapist, mother. You lie like a human question mark on the floor, looking up at me. I suspect we are both silently wondering the same thing.

What if I am not strong enough?

BITCHES AND BASTARDS

I open my new leather notebook and take the lid off my new blue pen.

I neatly write the title of today's topic at the top of the page.

Distraction skills.
I have started a DBT course (dialectical behaviour therapy). Apparently, it is going to help me learn and use new skills and strategies so that I can build a life that I think is worth living. I take notes while my new therapist recites anagrams. My notes are perfect. Keywords in blue and explanations in black. It all feels so manageable written down in colour-coded lists. I have been struggling for so long and all I needed to do was learn an anagram, stroke my dog, listen to soothing music and smell lavender. It all sounds so easy.

"Roxy, if the distraction skills don't work and you cannot resist the urges to hurt yourself, then you can inflict uncomfortable, shocking sensations on yourself."

I write a new title on a new page and then a new list:

- Hold ice
- Suck a lemon
- Draw red lines on wrist with a Sharpie

I want to tell her that there is no way a red Sharpie is going to stop me cutting. I open my mouth to speak and lift my head to look at her, but she is very busy ticking off the things she needs to tell me from her list. She isn't here to listen – her nose is stuck in the DBT what-to-say guide.

Hello, I am here.

I am being unfair. She is a kind and smart woman, but when I start to spiral, which is often, stroking my dog is not going to help. In fact, if I try to stroke my dog in that state, I will probably strangle her.

You tell me I need "tools in my toolbox". It is your favourite phrase. I hate that phrase. The therapist is giving me those tools, I know that, but you are so practical. I don't need more practical. I need to understand my brain and what is happening. As I sit here, I know what I should be talking to the therapist about: the fact that every time I look in a bathroom mirror, I see myself posing for photographs. At random moments, all the muscles in my body tense up because my head paints images that remind me of how disgusting I really am. I should tell her about the guilt I feel for running away and how I can't explain it because it feels like it was somebody else. Like I was possessed, but I wasn't. I should tell her that I miss the imaginary people because at least with them, I wasn't alone. I should say that I was blackmailed.

But I can't say any of this, so I'm a pretty useless patient. The poor therapist is trying her best.

When I become that spiralling mess, there is nothing anybody can say or do. I think I know that. I get angry and lash out at you, so it is best to leave me alone. But then, when I am alone, I get sad that I'm by myself. Nobody can win, I know that.

*

Now I am in another appointment with another doctor. A neurologist this time. She is going to check that there isn't a physical explanation for the hallucinations. I am a little excited that there might actually be a reason for all this craziness.

Early on in the appointment, it becomes clear that there isn't. I am just crazy.

So is this neurologist. She is completely nuts. She spends two hours giving me words of wisdom in her strong Argentinian accent with her arms flailing all over the place. She doesn't give me a brain scan.

"Girls are bitches and boys are bastards."

"Be good crazy, like me."

"Smile at people on the street."

"Help two people every day."

"Roxy, you are a baby with a good body."

"You made a mistake. It's in the past."

"Love yourself. Respect yourself."

"Look in the mirror and say, 'I am pretty.'"

The muscles in my body tense up, as if it is trying to block out these wise words.

I walk on to the street and I feel like I have been spun around in a washing machine for two hours. I also have this new feeling in my stomach. It is unfamiliar, which scares me. I think it might be the tiniest bit of hope.

Part 7

ICE ICE BABY

You cut yourself. It is March.

Really? After everything, you fucking cut yourself? No.

No. No. No. Since January we've been attempting to get you back on your feet with weekly trips to London for DBT. The days between appointments drag. We tried art therapy, but it wasn't for you; we tried yoga, but your mind needed more to chew on, not less. You went back to your wonderfully kind old maths teacher who taught you when you were 10, then we found a retired teacher to practise the triple sciences with you, and eventually the former head of maths who took your love of numbers to another level. This helped you believe that you weren't being completely left behind. Throughout February, generous souls have shared skills with you, kind people have walked and talked and cooked with you, your sisters have muted themselves around you. These heroes have helped you, backed you, rooted for you, loved you, and you thank them by taking a blade to your skin. It is not okay. Three long months tiptoeing through your recovery, and just like that, we tumble back to the bottom of the pit. I paw furiously through the drawer like a thief rummages for jewels – it's in here some-where. Shit, no it's not.

I can't remember where I've hidden all the bloody knives. Oh. Yes, I do. I grab one, yank up my shirt and fly towards you.

"Shall I cut myself, shall I, would that help, is that going to help?!" I am yelling now. I can't stop. It feels good to yell. I've been talking sotto voce for so long I don't recognize the sound of my voice. Even-keeled me. Calm. Considered. Cool. Now I have erupted.

You look pretty confused.

I fill the kitchen sink with freezing cold water. It's not cold enough, so I grab handfuls of ice and throw them in.

"You are not doing this any more!" I shout. "You are not doing it!"

Perhaps I am trying to drown out your thoughts, shout them down, scare them away. I am scared. I am so damn scared. Weeks of therapy, talking, training, walking, distraction techniques, breathing exercises, maths, collages, puzzles, guitar, I can't do it again, I can't go back and do it again. If it hasn't worked, then ….

I hold your hands in the water.

"It's not enough," you say.

"Take a breath," I insist. Then I plunge your face in the water.

You resurface.

"Again!" I shout.

Under you go.

You resurface. You take a huge gulp of air. Down you go.

I'm holding your hair up. I'm holding your head down. I could just hold you there … I step back.

We examine one another. Your face is crimson with cold.

"No more cutting," I say. "Do you understand?"

You nod.

"It ends now."

You nod again.

It doesn't end.

DUNKIN' KNIVES

"Feel the raisins in your palm. Move them slowly and focus your mind on the individual wrinkles."

This is bullshit. How are you not laughing at this lady?

Next, we are lying side by side on yoga mats doing breathing exercises. I cannot do them and they make me shake. The moment I start to breathe in and out on her command, my breathing quickens and I feel like I want to run as far away as I can from this weirdly warm shed. God, you are so good at this and I am so awful. Then she is guiding us through a 10-minute body scan. I really try, but suddenly I am thinking about my organs and blood vessels and how crazy it is that our bodies even work. There are so many things going on in our body and if one small thing stops working, then we die. Our nearest hospital is an hour away. I feel so fragile and my heart rate is increasing. I scramble around for things in my brain to distract me from this scary thought. The thing is, the teacher says that mindfulness will help me to control my brain and my thoughts, which I am so desperate to do. Imagine if my thoughts went where I told them to instead of the other way around.

So now I am at home, sitting at my desk, practising my mindfulness. First, I try to breathe in the right way. Breathe in for five seconds. Hold for five seconds. Breathe out for seven seconds. In for five seconds. Hold for five seconds. Out for seven seconds. In for five seconds. Hold for five seconds. Out for seven seconds. In for FUCK, SHIT, SHIT, FUCK, FUCK. I am now out of breath, a little dizzy, feeling way more uncomfortable than I did before, and cross with myself for being so useless. So I suck at breathing, that's great. I now try to focus completely on tracing the pattern around the edge of the desk with my mind. I am doing surprisingly well, but then the pattern reminds me of a tattoo, and I am thinking about what tattoo I would get and then I think I will get a puzzle piece and then I am thinking about the hours I spent doing puzzles and how totally pointless my life is and how I am the lamest teenager to ever walk on this planet. I decide that mindfulness is definitely not for me.

I go spend the day with my grandparents so that you can have some time for yourself. The house doesn't feel safe any more. It feels small and suffocating. This is where I hid from you when I sent all those photographs. My grandad's mirror. What kind of fucked-up child sends photographs taken in their grandad's mirror? Everything in this house reminds me of the photographs. The windowsill that I banged my head against and the lace throw that I hated. I pour all my energy into acting like I am okay and normal and sane. I ping the elastic band against my wrist. I want to hurt myself so badly.

"Don't do that, dear. You don't need to do that to yourself."

My grandma rests her hand against my wrist. Actually, I do need to do this. If I stop doing this, then there is a huge possibility that I go mental and take a knife to my wrist. The elastic band is better.

I do cut myself.

Then I tell you because I think that it is better to be open and honest. If you know, then I am less likely to do it again. I want you to know that I am really trying to use all the other skills. I am trying so hard to control my brain. This was just a mistake because I was tired and hurting. The photos invade my thoughts and it hurts. I think that if I try to tell you and explain, then we can have open, rational conversations about it.

You do not respond in a rational way.

You storm out of the room and I am confused.

Then you storm back in with a knife in your hand.

You lift up your T-shirt and hold the knife to your stomach.

"SHOULD I CUT MYSELF TOO? I AM IN PAIN TOO. SHOULD I SLICE AWAY AT MY STOMACH? IS THAT GOING TO HELP ANYTHING?"

My breathing starts to quicken and I feel myself losing control. You still have those same scary eyes. I have broken you. You are angry and you hate me for ruining your life. You are so caring towards me whenever there is somebody around, but as soon as we are alone, you switch. I know that I am ruining your life. My life is ruined too. I am sorry that I am not easy like your friends' children.

I am hyperventilating and starting to cry. How will we ever recover from this?

You take my sleeve and drag me over to the sink. You hold my head and dunk my face into freezing cold water. You do it over and over again.

The pain shoots from my cheeks and eyes into my body. It is the kind of pain that I crave when I hate myself this much.

You are dunking me fast, so I am struggling to breathe but I feel calm. Peaceful.

You really hate me. And I really hate me.

I wish that I could go away, get better, come back and be the daughter and sister that you guys want. There is nowhere for me to go. You took me out of hospital. You decided that you'd rather help me get better at home. You made that decision and now you are angry that I am here. Well, I am angry at you for not listening to me when I tried to tell you that I was struggling all those months ago, before everything about the photos came to light. I am furious that you didn't watch out for me after the photos came out. I am upset that you chose to not take any notice until it was way, way too late. I cannot believe that it took a social worker telling you to not leave me alone because I am extremely unwell before you decided that I was not just attention-seeking. I had to be actually psychotic before you decided to care. It didn't matter that I had gone through the most humiliating thing ever and was being bullied for it every single day. So yes, you are angry and I am angry and we have to contain that anger, otherwise nothing is going to get better.

STONES IN MY POCKETS

You are sitting on my dad's lap at Easter lunch. I don't know why. You like sitting on people's laps. I don't care – we're better than we were at Christmas and as far as I am concerned, that's a bloody miracle. You've joined lunch. You're chatty. You're not upstairs shouting at invisible people to go away.

"You're getting a bit heavy," says my dad.

"He means you've grown," I say, pre-empting your reaction, shutting him down. For fuck's sake, Dad.

I can see immediately it has landed badly with you.

"Pops said I was fat," you say later.

"He didn't …" It doesn't matter what I say. You've latched on. The thing is, there hasn't been a great deal to do other than eat, and the meds make you hungry. Eating breaks the monotony of an otherwise monotonous day. The walks we go on aren't exercise. We creep along, second by second, step by step, so yes, you've put on some weight.

You push the pasta on your plate to one side.

You refuse toast at breakfast.

"I'm not eating carbs," you say.

You start to cut out so many food groups there will be nothing left that you *can* have. After everything we've been through, we are not going to accidentally fall into the trap of an eating disorder.

Anorexia scares me. It killed a great friend's sister – total organ failure got her in the end. It has the lowest recovery rate of all the mental health illnesses: a third die. A third. That it can grab you and suck you under so easily terrifies me. A fad becomes a diet becomes a control issue becomes a death warrant. You said to me once that you thought you were in control of the voices, but then they took over and started to control you. I believe diets can do the same.

"We are not doing this!" I shout at you because once again, I am scared but I am also increasingly getting angry. Put the fucking matches down and stop, just stop, playing with fire. You despise me. I am your warden. A constant reminder that your life is not your own. I am the physical embodiment of all that has gone wrong. No wonder you despise me, but it is wearing me down. I am a nub of my former self. I need help. I need a break.

I had met Zizzi at a party when I first moved here. Like me, she is a blow-in from London. She's been here 20 years and knows everyone. She looks after people, from very old to very young and anyone in between. I think I am interviewing her. It becomes very apparent, very quickly, that she is interviewing me. For reasons I do not understand yet am eternally grateful for, she takes us on. Think Mary Poppins but with edge, attitude, some colourful language and a heart that is big enough for both of us. When she is in the house we are allowed to laugh. She is brilliant with your sisters too, picking them up from school and treating them to chips and gossip.

With neon glow sticks and a mountain of olives, the two of you go off laughing, dressed in Lycra, to the sports centre. I go for a walk, on my own, and it feels glorious. I stride out at a fast pace. It feels good. Soon I am running, it feels good to run and I normally hate running. But I run anyway, until I get to the sea.

I stand on the beach and look out to sea. We've come so far and been through so much. I am spent, there is nothing left in the tank. All I have to do is put some stones in my pockets, weigh myself down and walk into the sea. The water laps the shingle beach ridge, she is licking her lips, hungry. She could swallow me whole. I take a step back and wonder for the first time whether this might kill me. At the lowest moments of your recovery, I wonder if you want it to. I need help – not professional help, I'm still wary and suspicious of that – so I phone a friend.

Words spill out of me for over an hour, torrents of misery, fear and frustration. I am doing everything I can to help you get well, and all you do is lash out. She forwards me a letter. I sit on the beach and read it over and over.

Dear Parent,
This is the letter I wish I could write.
This fight we are in right now.
I need it. I need this fight.
I can't tell you this because I don't have the language for it and it wouldn't make sense anyway. But I need this fight badly. I need to hate you right now and I need you to survive it. I need you to survive my hating you and you hating me. I need this fight even though I hate it too. It doesn't matter what this fight is even about: curfew, homework, laundry, my messy room, going out, staying in, leaving, not leaving, boyfriend, girlfriend, no friends, bad friends, it doesn't matter.
I need to fight you on it and I need you to fight me back.
I desperately need you to hold the other end of the rope. To hang on tightly while I thrash on the other end – while I find the handholds and footholds in this new world I feel I am in. I used to know who I was, who you were, who we were. But right now, I don't. Right

now, I am looking for my edges, and I can sometimes only find them when I am pulling on you. When I push everything I used to know to its edge. Then I feel like I exist and, for a minute, I can breathe. I know you long for the sweeter kid that I was. I know this because I long for that kid too, and some of that longing is what is so painful for me right now.

I need this fight and I need to see that no matter how bad or big my feelings are, they won't destroy you or me. I need you to love me even at my worst, even when it looks like I don't love you. I need you to love yourself and me for both of us right now. I know it sucks to be disliked and labelled the bad guy. I feel the same way on the inside, but I need you to tolerate it and get other grown-ups to help you, because I can't right now. If you want to get all of your grown-up friends together and have a "surviving your teenager support group rage fest", that's fine with me. Or talk about me behind my back – I don't care. Just don't give up on me. Don't give up on this fight. I need it.

This is the fight that will teach me that my shadow is not bigger than my light. This is the fight that will teach me that bad feelings don't mean the end of a relationship. This is the fight that will teach me how to listen to myself, even when it might disappoint others.

And this particular fight will end. Like any storm, it will blow over and I will forget and you will forget. And then it will come back. And I will need you to hang on to the rope again. I will need this over and over, for years.

I know there is nothing inherently satisfying in this job for you. I know I will likely never thank you for it or even acknowledge your side of it. In fact, I will probably criticize you for all this hard work. It will seem like nothing you do will be enough. And yet, I am relying entirely on your ability to stay in this fight. No matter how much I argue. No matter how much I sulk. No matter how silent I get.

Please hang on to the other end of the rope. And know that you are doing the most important job that anyone could possibly be doing for me right now.

Love,

Your teenager

I adapt the image from the one in the letter, the one that demands I hold on no matter what. Instead, I tell myself that when the thrashing gets so severe as to threaten to maim me or pull me in, I am allowed to let the rope out just a little. I allow myself a bit of space. I cannot help you if I am down there with you – so I mustn't fall and I mustn't let go – but I don't have to take every thrashing either. I go home. I can do this. I can keep holding on even though every muscle aches with the strain of it. It is not easy and it is not quick. Sometimes you get tantalizingly close to the top, almost out, and other times you are thrown back in, and as the rope rips through my fingers, it burns. But I hold on and slowly, slowly, oh so slowly, you start to climb out of that deep, dark well.

CLUBBERCISE

"Stop looking so fucking sorry for yourself, Roxy. Life is not that bad."

Zizzi is not amazing at sympathy, which is probably a good thing, but it still pisses me off. I glare at her as she speeds around another corner. You have decided that you cannot manage me by yourself, so you are paying somebody else to help you. I was hurt at first. It is your job to look after me, but instead you want to go back to your old life – filled with yoga, Pilates and drinking coffee – and palm me off to some stranger. Luckily, that stranger ended up being Zizzi. She is my fairy godmother and is like nobody I have ever met before. Twice a week, she comes into our kitchen like a whirlwind of light and fun. When she is here, we can breathe, and nothing seems that bad.

She is straightforward, there is no bullshit. She doesn't treat me like I am sick. She gossips with me, makes me feel like a teenager again. She tells me wildly inappropriate stories about people from my school. I don't know how much is strictly true, but I laugh for the first time in a long time. She has clearly lived so much of life; she has met crazy people and she reminds me how small my world is at the moment. Zizzi becomes my family. She is my other mother. She gives me everything you can't and vice versa. She gives me perspective. She makes me feel so normal and special at the same time. She completely gets me.

We are in the car on the way to the supermarket. She is driving so fast around every corner, it is a miracle we are still alive. These outings to the supermarket are a hugely valuable break from the monotony of our kitchen. It is more of a social occasion than a chore. Zizzi is wearing a huge fur jacket with gold hoops and black-heeled boots. She looks incredible. She always looks incredible. She knows almost everybody who works in Tesco by name, and those she doesn't she calls "darling". She has this way of making everybody feel a bit special, even if it is a 30-second conversation. She tells the lady stacking shelves that her hair looks incredible and asks if she is using a new product. She tells the man behind the counter that he has lost weight and looks great. We stop off at the chip shop on the way home. She completely goes to town flirting with the guy who works there. I just stare at her in awe. She makes it all look so easy and grace-ful. Everybody she speaks to, she leaves them smiling.

Zizzi has somehow persuaded me to go to a Clubbercise class at the local gym. Apparently, there is no excuse to be fat and we both need to get out of the house and lose some weight. I am the youngest here by at least 50 years and definitely the slimmest. Somehow I have ended up spending my Thursday night in a dark studio dancing to bad 1990s music with glow sticks in my hand. Weirdly, I don't feel like a loser. When I am with Zizzi, I can walk around without wanting to be invisible. I am smiling properly for the first time in a really long time. I hop from side to side, watching my glow sticks change colour. The front wall of the room is a mirror, but it doesn't scare me tonight. I am smiling and clothed. After the class, we decide that we've earnt a snack, so we scoff an entire pot of olives in the Tesco car park.

Zizzi is so different from everybody around here and is just so confident in her own individuality. She helps me grow and get better. She won't stand for any self-pity and she teaches me to take responsibility.

"Own your shit, Roxy."

She changes my life.

I decide to log on to Instagram for the first time in months today. I still don't have a phone, so I use your computer. I feel sick scrolling through. There was a party last night and everyone is posting photos. I try to laugh at how they are all wearing the exact same black dress, they have the same hair and the same make-up and the same shoes. I try to smirk at the lack of individuality, but honestly, I just feel sad and left out. I wish I was posing in those photos, wearing that black dress and those shoes and straightening my hair. It is an unwanted reminder that while my life has been put on hold, everyone else's is carrying on without me. It seems obvious, but I had sort of forgotten that there is still a world outside of this kitchen. I seem to be going backwards, and everybody else is growing up. My other aching thought is that these straight-haired skinny girls in black dresses are going to want nothing to do with this frizzy-haired mess of a person.

I begin teaching myself maths GCSE out of sheer boredom. I need something in this miserable, repetitive life. Then I set myself the challenge of sitting the exam this coming summer, a year early – I'll still only be 14. The numbers become my mindfulness. They work for me. Their exactness is so clear. The problems are solvable and they take extreme focus. My mind that seems unable to handle most real-life things can handle maths. It soothes me. I can throw myself into a page of working, and the feeling when I get to the final answer is amazing. Most of the time my brain feels so useless. It seems to do everything wrong and tricks me all the time and then suddenly, we can work together to solve these really hard problems. Two amazing maths teachers give me their time. They must know what I did and I cannot imagine what they think of me. I know that they care and they know that I am grateful, but we don't have to say any of that. Instead, we talk about quadratics. They remind me how much my brain can actually do.

*

We are having tea with the wife of my old headmaster, the one who scooped me up when I first went to boarding school. She has cancer and her last round of chemo is this week. She gives me some books to read and we talk about records. We compare funny stories about how people treat you when you're sick. We laugh about side effects. She tells me that we are both ill but we are both going to get better. She talks to me like mental illness is exactly the same as her physical illness and there is nothing to be ashamed of. She doesn't get better.

I sit up panting and sweating. My window and curtains are closed. It was just a bad dream, another bad dream. I have that same dream every night for months: I am in my bed and I see myself sitting on the windowsill with my legs hanging out. The girl I see is pale. She is being tortured by loud, invisible people who shout. She looks back at me; her eyes are crazy and chaotic. I shout out to her, but as I do, she pushes herself forward off the windowsill. Then I wake up. It is the same, every night.

FLY-TIPPING

Someone has dumped a big black bin bag in the middle of the lane. The bin bag moves. It's you. I start running. There is a party for your year group that night and we have talked, over and over, about the pros and cons of you going. You are fitter, stronger, happier. Its halfway through April and you've worked so hard on your maths that you'll be sitting your GCSE even though you aren't at school. I want to reward that effort by letting you go because I fear the impact of you missing out on yet another highlight of your year could be a genuine threat to your recovery. But now, as I stand over you, crumpled on the tarmac, I realize the fear of going is also a genuine threat to your recovery. I am back on that tightrope. The one that feels like a blade beneath my feet. One wrong step, and …

It is pure luck a car didn't come around that corner and kill you, but your luck may soon run out. I can hear a car in the distance. You won't get up. I drag you to the side of the road and we sit there and watch the car pass terrifyingly close. Of course the party is out of the question, what was I thinking? I need to get you to London to see the therapist. Zizzi offers to take you to the station, but as soon as you two leave, I question my own sanity. Two pressing thoughts: How can I let you travel by train on your own? Months and months have passed and still you're a risk to yourself, all because of a party? And secondly, if you miss that party, the risk to you is even greater. I call the DBT therapist in London you are still regularly seeing and we talk through the options. You have told her nothing of these moments, I am always filling her in. God knows what you two talk about. I wish I knew, but as ever, she tells me nothing. I second-guess everything even though I have a professional on the line. I make a decision and phone Zizzi.

"Come back," I say. "It's not safe." She agrees but she is also pleased; she really wants you to go to the party.

"Life has to be lived," she says. You have to start living it. I think you go to make her proud. I take you to the party, never feeling sure whether it is the dumbest thing to do, the least bad option or courageous on both our parts – and truthfully, we will never know. I join other mothers at a pizzeria, but as ever I feel completely dislocated from the chat. My normal is not their normal. When you emerge, you seem fine and I pray you've had fun. You see me and stumble. Are we back to that too?

Use your words. It's a refrain I used when you were little. It still applies.

I know that re-entry to your old life is going to prove very, very hard and is going to require the patience of a saint. I am no saint. Thankfully, I have found people to help me help you rebuild your life. I was able to carry you when you were ill, but recovery takes a village. Anyone in our position must find their own.

Without a doubt, Zizzi remains the chieftain of ours.

BIN BAG

A stone sticks sharply into my cheek and another one into my temple. My head is rested painfully on the black tar road and there is a pothole next to my arm. The black rain jacket I'm wearing flaps and blows in the wind. My legs cannot carry me any more; they are too tired, I am too tired. I can't go back to the kitchen. This is not living. I still spend most of my time with you and it is clear you deeply dislike me. You always have, but now your eyes are tinted with hatred. I am ruining your life and our family. Of course I know that. Nobody in our house is happy and that is my fault.

I am supposed to be going to a party tomorrow, but I can't do it. I am the freak that everybody thinks I am. I can't speak to people, I freeze up. I can't just dance and have fun – I would feel like an imposter. My right arm has gone dead under the weight of my body.

Move, I tell my body. *Get off the ground.*

I am too tired to move, and my arms and legs won't do what I tell them. I can't face the way people at the party will look at me like I have escaped from a mental hospital. Technically, I am not ill any more – there are no hallucinations, the medication has worked. I should be better. I don't feel better. I am desperately sad and anxious all the time. I have no friends, no plans and my obsessive brain controls me. I am going to have to build my life again from the beginning. Knowing this is suffocating me. It has chained me to rock bottom because the climb back up seems so impossible. At the core of all of this, I am the problem.

I hear a car engine nearby. You run over and scoop me up. I feel a pang of sadness; it could've all been over, just like that. I don't know if I am suicidal. I don't have a plan to kill myself.

I don't have rope or a gun. I have my pot of pills but I haven't collected enough yet. I think I might want my life to be over, though. I cannot visualize a future for myself. If I try to envision my life a year from now, I just see black nothingness. I think maybe I am not supposed to have a future. I am stuck and next year doesn't exist. Anyway, if my life is just going to be you, me, our kitchen, naked photos, pain, fear, sleeplessness, then I am not sure that I want a future to exist.

You somehow persuade me to go to the party.

You're right, I think, *if I don't go, then the self-loathing will set me back weeks. What is the worst that can happen? I am showing my face and proving that I'm not a freak.*

I say this to myself on repeat that night so that I don't go hide in the toilet. I am standing between two skinny girls with perfectly straightened hair for photographs. We are pretending we are all friends, but I know I am only there because you've organized everything, as usual, with the mothers. I hate my outfit; I look fat. I am wearing a huge baggy jumpsuit that covers everything. I am not a slut, I am not a psycho. My arms look fat and my hair is a tangled, frizzy mess. The girls are trying to be nice and one offers me her spare dress. God, I wanted to wear it so badly, but her mum said to me:

"Everybody is expecting you to wear a dress like that, so don't do it."

I am not a slut, I am not a psycho. I don't really dance at the party because I'm not wearing a bra. People are nice and they smile, but they also have put a barrier up. They are kind, but they keep me at a distance. Some of these people were my friends once upon a time, but they all disappeared. Everybody here is trying to be so grown-up. Tiny dresses, suits, six-inch stilettos, pretending to be drunk from the one miniature bottle of vodka that they hid in their bras. A girl I know runs up to me and brags that she has already made out with seven boys, and asked me how many I had kissed. I don't think that I will ever be able to do that again. I used to find it so easy. Now, the idea of somebody touching me, of a boy getting close enough to me for us to kiss – it makes me feel sick.

I pretend not to notice that the girls I arrived with drop me as soon as they find the group that they would rather be seen with. Or that when I dance with a group of girls, they slowly make the circle smaller and smaller until I have been subtly choreographed out of it. I am left awkwardly jiggling around by myself until I think that I might cry. They are right, of course. I have no right to be here. This morning, I was a bin bag in the road and now I am pretending that I should be at a party. I take a puff of a cigarette that someone passes me. I cough – so embarrassing. I used to be able to do that. I used to be able to do all of this and I loved it, and it ruined me. I have nothing to add to conversations and I don't have the confidence to dance like nobody is watching. I kill some time sitting in the bathroom because this party is exhausting. Finally, it is over. I hated every second of it but I'm still glad I went. It is a step towards going back to real life and I wouldn't have been able to forgive myself if instead I had spent another night sitting in our kitchen.

I walk down the steps out of the venue and spot you with all the other mothers, who are waiting eagerly for their perfect little darling daughters. I have used every molecule of energy in my body to be okay for the past few hours. As soon as I see you, I let go of the final drop of strength that was holding me together. I need you to catch me. I need you to know that although I survived this party, I am not better.

You are still angry at me for lying in the road.

THE MOTHERLODE

You are going back to school. A whole term ahead of schedule. I am not surprised. You've always been an outlier, and you've always liked to prove people wrong. The psychiatrist has recommended new medication to help you with the transition. You will come off the antipsychotic drug and move to an antidepressant, which, at a certain dosage, acts as an anti-anxiety medication. The key is the dosage. I don't like messing with meds like this, but I also want you to be able to look over the horizon without seeing enemy in the grass. Dr B also wants us to begin family therapy. I have only agreed because of two things. Firstly, the family therapist is part of Dr B's team and therefore has spoken to him and your therapist in detail and knows the backstory, the situation and all the bits and pieces that we are not allowed to know about because of client confidentiality. I am hopeful that finally, finally, someone will tell us what this is all about, because I still don't know.

The second reason is more complicated. You have two parents, you've had two parents since birth, so I am a bit sick of taking all the heat and flak. The complication is that you are refusing to attend if your dad is there.

"Two against one," you say. "Dad always takes your side."

I won't go if he's not there. You won't go if he is. A perfect catch-22.

Your dad and I decide to go together to learn what we can. We sit opposite her. The woman looks like she should be running a sweet shop in the Village of the Year. She has a quaint face. She sits neatly on the armchair opposite with a thick file on her lap. She keeps asking me questions. I look at your dad. I've really had enough of this. I have been searching out answers and taking on responsibility for your behaviour since you were four.

She asks me another question.

I look at your dad. I've told him that this prolonged attack on me has to stop. I've told him I fear it might kill me. I've told him I fear I might break.

He answers for me, backs me up, explains and encourages her to understand the extraordinary complexity of being needed and hated in equal measure – but the thing is, it is still about me. Not us. Never him. How come? He is hardly baggage-free. I don't understand. For two hours, they talk about you and me, almost as if I weren't there. Then she looks at me, her head cocked to one side.

"So, do you feel like you can put your arm around her and give her a hug?"

I'm sorry, what? Tears of disappointment and anger sting my eyes. That's what you've got? A hug? Haven't you been listening. I am living with a tyrannical baby, a prickly pear, a whirling dervish, a rag doll. I want to tell her to fuck off, but I know that will look bad on my record and I guess, since we are in family therapy, I am still on thin ice.

"Can you just tell her you love her?"

There it is. The motherlode. I am the missing piece of the puzzle.

Everyone is telling me to love you unconditionally, but sometimes it feels like I am in an abusive relationship where you get to say and do anything you want and I just have to take it. I wouldn't take this from a boyfriend or friend, do I really have to take it from my child?

Hold on, hold on, just hold on.

*

I am sitting in a script meeting with a director and he is flicking through his iPad to find a photo of an actress he likes for a part. I can't place her. Swipe, swipe, swipe, erect penis, swipe, swipe,

swipe. I stare at the screen. He says nothing. I say nothing. We sit there. He closes the iPad. Some men are dicks and I am a coward, the bystander I tell my daughters not to be. I need something good to come of all this.

The school email me – would I write a piece for mental health awareness week? Hang on, you're going back in mental health awareness week? Full of talks about how good the school is at dealing with the mental health of their students? Everyone looking at you in assembly? We delay your return by a week and I write the piece. I call it "When You Lose It".

"I think Roxy took a blade from the building site."

It's Zizzi on the line. She's been looking after you while I've been in London. You and she had gone for an outing to see the house we are building. We need a permanent home and have decided that a new-build is the answer. It will be well-insulated, eco, warm and light. We've designed a space for a bed in a room off ours if things don't get better. We want you to feel safe and secure, not alarmed by creaking doors and the eerie cry of wind spiralling down chimney stacks.

"I saw her looking at it. Then when she was back in the car, I said I had left my scarf, went back in, and the Stanley knife had gone. It's a blow. Also …," she continues, "you should change your password on the computer, she's been reading your emails."

Six months in and still I can't get complacent, I can't relax, I can't take my eye off the ball, not even for a second – and yet, you're back at school? The mind boggles that we are still balancing so precariously on a knife-edge.

*

You are hiding in a bush near the sports shed. I am here to take you to an appointment with the mindfulness teacher. It's part of the scaffolding of your new week: alongside lessons, you will continue with the bi-weekly trips to London to see the therapist and you will exercise with Zizzi. In the afternoons, you come home and work through stacks of past GCSE maths papers. The appointments are the pitons that will help you climb out of the well. Small footholds that we hammer into the slimy dark wall.

You didn't like mindfulness but you liked the teacher.

"She understands me," you say, with that edge in your voice that I have learnt to live with. It means *not like you*.

"She's kind." *Not like you.* I tense and take the punch. I put my arm around you.

"I am really pleased you like her." Then I tense again, waiting for the look, the undercut jab. *Not like you.* Sticks and stones, babygirl, sticks and stones.

But now you won't come out of the bush. You say the woman scared you. Now you don't like her.

"What are you talking about?"

"I'm not going back," you whimper.

"What happened?"

You shake your head. The bush rustles.

I call the woman myself. "What happened? I can't get her in the car."

"Sorry," she says, "client confidentiality." What a crock of shit.

I realize that pitons, those precious footholds, also damage the surface they are hammered into. They create chips and splinters and since they are malleable, they also deform to match the shape of the void they are trying to fill. We are slaves to this system because we have nothing else to hang on to – and make no mistake, it is a long, lonely, strenuous climb.

PREGNANCY OR THE FLU

It is my first day back at school and I have just started a new medication. It is making me drowsy and groggy. Everything feels numbed and my brain is slow.

"Roxy, long time no see. Have you had the flu?"

I laugh nervously because what on Earth am I meant to say? I really try to concentrate in lessons, but the words swim around on the page and don't stay in the correct order. I feel stupid. In maths, I try to concentrate on the topics. I am good at maths; I have taught myself all of this. I am actually ahead, and yet I cannot concentrate on the numbers. The girls on the table behind me chatter and laugh and whisper.

They aren't talking about you, Roxy. Come on, it is in your head.

Their whispers and laughs make me paranoid and anxious. The whispers float all around me and I cannot focus on the maths. Maths makes sense. People do not.

"Roxy, how's the baby?"

"Roxy, long time no see!"

"Roxy, any more photos to share with us?"

I really thought that people would've forgotten, moved on, found something more interesting to talk about. Those stupid photos will never disappear. They will float around, phone to phone, group chat to group chat, boy to boy. How do I look these people in the eye? How do I expect anybody to look at me and not see the photos?

I don't go into the cafeteria any more. I'm too scared. Instead, I eat soup in the teachers' kitchen. I've cut out carbs because I am fat. I eat my pea soup alone and I don't go to assembly.

The boys are here. They seem to be everywhere. They are happy and thriving. I do fall into slumps of self-pity. I hate that those boys live their lives normally and nothing bad happens to them. I hate that Liz probably hasn't thought twice about what she did. I hate that we still live in a time where the young vulnerable girl is the one who pays. Then I hate myself because I know that I did this. I could've stopped all of this from happening. I hate you and I love you, but most of all I need you – and then I hate myself for needing you. See, it is messy and chaotic and a constant battle with my own head and a sun salutation is not going to fix any of that.

A week later, I am hiding in a bush. It is Wednesday lunchtime and I am supposed to be going to a mindfulness session. I have continued seeing the mindfulness lady. We do more talking than mindfulness. She is kind and gentle, she listens to me and acknowledges how shit this is. She doesn't offer practical solutions. Her shed was a warm sanctuary for me. A valuable escape from our kitchen.

Then last week, she went crazy. Completely lost it. She has always spoken openly about herself and she clearly has her own issues.

I am losing weight now because of my strict no-carb diet. In our session last week, she told me that I am losing too much weight.

"Your face looks too thin."

She started to cry. Between sobs, she told me that she stopped eating when she was younger.

"Roxy, I wanted to die. I don't want you to die."

Tears streamed down her face and she begged me not to turn out like her. Between gulps for air, she told me that life is hard, life is so hard. I couldn't look at her. She was a mess, completely broken. I sound uncompassionate, I know, but I can't handle it. I can't go back and face her. I really like her, but I am barely staying above water and I just can't watch somebody else lose it.

So now I am hiding in a bush.

I take Zizzi on a tour of our new house, which is a building site. She is not in a good mood. Ranting about absolutely everything. We are standing in my room and I notice a small silver blade glistening on the windowsill. I want to go over to it, cradle it in my hands. I want to stroke my finger over the edge of the blade. I don't do this because I am better now, I am "fixed", and that is not the sort of thing that fixed people do. As we walk around the house, I can hear the blade calling me – "Come get me, come get me." I clench my teeth and try to focus on something else. This is a time when mindfulness would probably come in handy, but I still suck at that. Eventually, I cannot take it any more, and I tell Zizzi I am going to the bathroom. I run to the windowsill and stuff the blade into my sleeve. The cold metal touching my wrist sends a warm shiver up my arm and all over my body. I am not going to do anything with the blade; I am better – I just want to feel the strength of it. We are about to drive away, but Zizzi has forgotten something in the house, then we go home. A few days later, I have hidden the blade and have resisted all temptations to use it. I am proud of myself. You call me, angry because Zizzi told you I took the blade. I have no idea how she even noticed. I thought I was so subtle. She has "thrown me under the bus", one of her favourite expressions and I am mad at her. I thought she was on my side. I tell you I haven't used it or anything but I understand that you have no reason to believe me. How am I supposed to explain that just having it hidden under my sleeve is enough? That I am working so hard to get better and this was a compromise. I get rid of the blade and I feel weak.

*

My maths teacher has asked a difficult question. Nobody is answering. I know the answer, but I don't know if I can speak out loud in front of all these people. I slowly raise my hand just above my head, sort of praying that the teacher doesn't notice. He makes eye contact with me and I wonder if he sees a smart student or me in my underwear. I answer the question. I taught myself this topic when I was off school. I did it – I spoke in front of the whole class, I drew attention to myself and didn't freak out about it. It feels amazing.

I have rebuilt a few friendships. They are intense, though, and I can only really handle it when it is just me with one other person. As soon as I am in a group, I have no idea what to say. I am not witty or funny and I am too slow. It is still nice to have a couple of friends that I can talk to. It is a step, but I am still a long way from being fun again.

I decide that I am going to take part in sports day. I was always the fastest girl in my year, but up until today, I was pretty sure I was going to find a reason to skip the race. Now I am here, standing at the starting line in these tiny, skintight running shorts and school vest that shows half my bra, and I am about to sprint in the 200-metre race past the entire school. I might as well be naked.

It's nothing they haven't all seen before.

I am just going to run as fast as I can and deal with the chattering voice in my head telling me that everybody was laughing about the photos after the race. I run and I win and nobody mentions the pictures.

I am still not eating any carbohydrates, so I have lost all the weight I gained from sitting in our kitchen for months. I like what I look like, so I am experimenting with going back to my old clothes instead of the oversized jumpers I have been living in. I am going to the school summer rock concert with a few people. I am wearing some tight jeans and a see-through mesh top. I see Zizzi, she's there to support me, but I dismiss her with a small smile; I know how rude it is as I do it. Dan and his band are the main act in the concert. He sings and plays the guitar confidently; he isn't embarrassed at all – there is no shame or guilt there. How can I be standing here cheering and dancing and oohing and aahing with all these girls?

The girl next to me nudges my side and whispers, "I mean, he is just so attractive."

I feel that warm feeling of pride rise up through my body. It is a feeling that I recognize and am terrified of. Why am I here? I shouldn't be here. How do I still think he is attractive? Why am I wearing these tight clothes and still wondering if he has noticed? Not just him even – any boys, I'm wondering if *any* boys have noticed. How is this still a part of me? After everything that has happened, how?

SWEETIE JAR

Zizzi makes the olive oil concoction; we make you drink it and I put my fingers down your throat. I know when the pills are out because I can see the misshapen red plasticky coating of the fast-acting ibuprofen glowing bright against the grass. We are hiding in the back of the garden so your little sister can't see. In your hand you are still clutching a plastic sweet pot. A cartoon face smiles at me. I know that pot. It comes from the sweet dispenser machine in the pub near my mother's house. You must have been stashing these for ages. You retch a final time. Nothing else comes up but a mollusc of slimy bile. Zizzi and I stare, perplexed, at one another over your head. She is on your side. She is on my side too.

"What the fuck?" she mouths.

I roll my eyes. What the fuck, indeed. This does not make sense. You've been getting steadily better, stronger, able to stand on your own two feet. You survived the summer term back at school, part-time I know and well-supervised, but back. You'd exceeded Dr B's expectations, you'd started making new friends, you'd even sat your maths GCSE, a year early! Now what? Do you need your stomach pumping? It's the 2nd of July and we are back discussing A&E? "I'm sorry," you say over and over. "I don't know why I did that. I'm sorry." I really hope your sister is watching telly.

"What was in there, Roxy?"

"Just a few pills."

"How many?"

"I don't know."

I count four, maybe five red jellies in the grass and try and calculate how fast "fast-acting" means. They are deformed. Your stomach acid has already started work on the outer shell. I haven't a clue what I am doing. Why did you take them? You'd been to a birthday party last night. You'd looked great and had fun. I don't understand. When am I going to understand? *Hold on, hold on ...*

"Try and remember what you took."

"It was paracetamol and ibuprofen."

Zizzi and I set you on the grass and huddle. Team talk.

"She'd have to take handfuls of those to kill herself," she says. My thoughts are racing.

"She can't have taken handfuls. Handfuls she'd remember. I don't think she's taken enough to kill herself," I say.

We look back at you. You're alert, in a stunned, "what the fuck have I done" way. You're not slurring your words. You look scared, though. I think you've scared yourself. Call me the perennial optimist, but I think maybe this is a good thing.

SALT AND OLIVE OIL

"Mummy, I've done something stupid."

I do know that it was stupid, but 10 minutes ago it felt like the only option. My little sweet pot has sat patiently in my bedside table for months, slowly filling up with painkillers, lorazepam, risperidone – anything I could subtly steal. I promise you that I wasn't planning this. They were a comfort, but I wasn't planning to take them. It was just like holding the blade in my coat pocket. It soothed me.

Today, I very calmly took out the sweet pot and poured the collection of pills down my throat.

I was at a party last night and I had an amazing time. I wore a tight black miniskirt and mesh top. I straightened my hair and wore make-up. I got drunk and talked to everybody. I made jokes about why I had disappeared so that people felt at ease with me. I smoked cigarettes and danced and held my friend's hair up while she puked.

So this makes no sense.

"Mummy, please can I talk to you?"

"No. I am doing something with Reva."

I stand here waiting. I can't say this in front of Reva, not after everything I have already put my sisters through.

Reva leaves.

"I've taken some pills, Mummy. Nothing serious, just a few ibuprofen and paracetamol. I just thought that I should tell you."

"How many?"

"I don't know why I did it. I don't know how many. I'm sorry."

You look at me with the same cold eyes. I am too dramatic for you; you hate unnecessary drama. You call Zizzi and of course, she knows exactly what to do.

I stick my fingers down my throat, but nothing comes. Then you do it with your fingers and still nothing.

I gulp back a cup of salt water and cry. Nothing happens.

Then Zizzi hands me a cup of olive oil and tells me to drink. I drink.

I am violently sick.

I am sad to lose all those little pills that have kept me company for so many months.

I can't explain it to either of you. I just had to take those pills. I cannot put the feeling into words. There isn't a way to describe it, it was just there.

I can now try to explain. It's taken years and it still doesn't make complete sense, but I have an idea of what that feeling was. I had an incredible time the night before. I wasn't sick any more, I was better. I was the girl I used to be. Except I didn't want to be the girl I used to be and I wasn't better. I wasn't better because I was the girl I used to be. Scared, anxious, my brain working a million miles a minute, always, constantly, switched on to max. If it wasn't the illness any more, then it was me. I was the problem. That thought terrified me more than being ill ever terrified me. When I was ill, I was other. Now that I was well, I was me. So now the insurmountable, daunting task of fixing me lay ahead – and that was all, there was nothing else. I couldn't go back to being the party girl in the short skirt using hair straighteners, but I couldn't go forward either. I was in no man's land. I had been deconstructed, left in pieces, without the ability, energy or desire to reconstruct my life. How could I rebuild myself? I couldn't. So I took the pills.

Thankfully, I couldn't do that either.

Part 8

HORNET'S NEST

Another September rolls around and here we are again. Third time lucky, I think, as I stand in the garden with a cup of coffee, my dog and a friend's puppy playing at my feet. Above me is the windowsill you sat on less than a year ago. We are a million miles from that place, I know. I hope I know. Still, only two of my children went back to school this morning. You are in Manchester with your dad at a work photo shoot. You cannot return to your old life, nor can you see a way to build a new life here. I believe you can fix what is broken. You believe what is broken cannot be fixed. Not here. Not in situ. Not with all the boys still walking around, their lives uninterrupted.

"But they've left," I plead.

"The teachers haven't," you reply.

"Some amazing teachers really tried to help."

"My maths teacher saw the photos."

I realize it is tough facing the friends who abandoned you, seeing the women who once crossed the road but now offer you thin, inauthentic smiles. Walking through town feels like walking through a minefield. Any second, we can turn a corner and – boom. We are left picking up body parts. Still, I am worried. Your solution is a sixth-form college in another city, living in student accommodation, and compressing two years of study into one. Isn't it all a bit much?

Your dad and Dr B strongly agree with you. I am outnumbered. So we sign you up. When we tell the school, the headmaster replies to the news with a few lines, including: *I am personally very worried about the idea of college.* Me too. Perhaps if he'd been more concerned about your recovery you would still be safely under my roof. I felt he gave up on you pretty damn fast. You are such a smart, talented girl, I don't understand why he doesn't fight harder for you, but he doesn't. And so once again, four of us will be in one place, and one of us – you – will be somewhere else.

I tell your dad that I will not be doing mercy missions to pick you up when the wheels fall off. I am not a supporter of this decision and am handing the baton of responsibility over to him. He goes up and down to London, he passes through the city where you will live, it's up to him now. He assures me the wheels won't fall off. He is an extraordinarily positive person, yet I am dumbfounded by his attitude. We've been carrying you and now you're just going to skip off, solo, into the sunset? He and I argue for the first time since I was called into that office a year ago. Zizzi has said to me since she thought it was a miracle we stayed together. The stress feels unbearable at times, but we figured out early that we had to figure this out together or we would fail. It becomes a lot harder now that we don't agree on how to proceed. Friction causes cracks.

"Ow!"

A bee has flown into my hair and stung me. It stings me again. Not a bee. I can hear frantic buzzing now – a wasp is stuck in my mad curly hair. I try and flick it out when I see a large hornet on my thigh. It stings me through my leggings. I drop the coffee cup.

"OW!"

There is also a hornet on the puppy.

"Shit!"

The buzzing becomes more of a whine – high-pitched, urgent. Another sting to the head and I realize I'm in big trouble. I strip off my leggings. They are under my T-shirt. I strip that off too. I try and get them out of my hair, running frantically around the garden, shouting every time I get another sting. Eventually,

I stick my head under a tap. My scalp is on fire. Perhaps I am going to die. What a fucking ridiculous way to go. They will find me in old grey pants with a couple of dead dogs … I start to shake. For the second time in my life, I dial 999. Twelve hornet stings and a trip in the back of an ambulance later, I have a chance to reflect. You are starting your new life. By some miracle, I am not dead. I would like to restart mine.

By the time I am released, somehow your dad is there to take me home. I am wearing his dressing gown and fall into his bear hug. We feel very lucky. We will make sure those cracks don't turn into chasms. We have to take care of each other a bit now, and we have to take care of your sisters a lot, they've had a long year with a lost sister and less than half a mother. You will have to learn to take care of yourself, regulate your own emotions and forgive yourself.

How is this going to work?

You're only fifteen. Still so young and yet older than your years.

ONE YEAR ON

I have managed one month in my new school. It is a sixth-form college, but they are letting me cram my GCSEs into one year. It isn't even really a year - I have two terms to learn two years' worth of content. I didn't want to run away again, I really wanted to go back to my old school and not let them win. I just couldn't sit in maths lessons knowing that my teacher had seen those photos. Everyone had seen those photos. I am living in the most depressing student accommodation. It is a square room with a small window, a single bed, a desk and about 1 metre square of floor space. I am in a new city where nobody knows what I did, nobody thinks I am crazy and nobody thinks I am a slut. It is exactly what I wanted. A fresh start, anonymity. But I am so, so alone.

Every day is one year since something happened. A year since the prostitute call. A year since the photos came out. A year since I first cut myself. A year since I ran away. A year since I sat out the window. A year since I was put in hospital. My brain slips back and forth between now and then. One minute, I am sitting in a French lesson and the next I am back with the angels, and they are talking. I can't control where my mind takes me, and it keeps taking me back. I don't cut any more, or make myself sick. I don't eat carbs and I go for runs. I make sure that there isn't a second in the day when I don't have anything to do. I study solidly until I take a sleeping pill at 9 p.m. Then I watch one episode of TV and draw cubes on a scrap piece of paper. Then I fall asleep. Sleep is still a scary place. I usually see myself sitting out the window or a man hanging from my ceiling. The same recurring dreams.

I go days without speaking to another person other than my teachers. I avoid any common areas in the college – I am not ready for people my age yet. I wear very baggy clothes. Big sweatshirts and jeans that are way too big for me. I am not ready for people to see my body again. Dad comes to have lunch with me and I just explode. I talk non-stop at him for an hour and then he leaves. I sent him a text yesterday trying to explain that I know I'm not very good company and don't listen to what he has to say, but it is only because when I see him, I haven't had a conversation with anybody in days.

You and I don't really speak. We have gone from spending every second of every day together to barely being able to be in the same room. I sometimes call you when I am overwhelmingly sad, you say the wrong thing, and then we don't speak. I know that you are relieved to not have me in the house. When I was 10, I ran away to boarding school and now I've done it again. How fucked is it that we cannot live under the same roof? You don't miss me. I miss you so much. I am back in the place where I need you and I hate myself for needing you and I hate you for not being the person I need. I don't think we can come back from this. I think that you will forever blame me for the past year and I will forever blame you for not being the person that I could come to way back at the beginning, when all of this could have been prevented. I am sad about a lot of what has happened, but our relationship is the thing that breaks me the most. After our bad phone calls, I go for long walks through the city listening to Joni Mitchell's 'Both Sides Now' on repeat. When I was younger, you would play it on the piano and I would sing. It makes me cry a lot.

I didn't really live with my sisters when they were younger. Then we spent two years in the same house; during the first year, I was rude and completely uninterested in their lives. During the second, I was sick and sucked up every molecule of happiness in our lives. I don't blame any of you for not being sad that I am gone, but living with that feeling is eating me up.

*

It is 3 a.m. and there is a man standing at the end of my bed. He arrived during a nightmare about a plane crash, but he has stayed. I am fully awake now, but he came out of my dream and now he won't go away. I don't turn the light off and I am scared to close my eyes. He is thin and tall and his skin has a yellow tint. He doesn't say anything and he doesn't move, he just stands there and stares. I am obviously not going to tell anybody about this.

I am not ill. I am not ill. I am better. I am fixed.

I have recovered from my mental illness and now I am in the "putting your life back together" stage. I am supposed to be the person that went through something horrible, came out the other side, and has put my life back together. I want to be that person, but there is a man standing at the end of my bed.

HEADBANGER

Your hatred of me has risen like a phoenix out of the ashes of your life. They say time heals, but it also hurts. With every passing month that you get further from the moment your life imploded, you simultaneously lose more time not able to live the life you should be living. The more time you spend healing, the more time it costs you to heal. It's a horrendous conveyor belt taking you on to another anniversary of another miserable event that you can't undo and you can't escape and you can't outrun. I have clawed back the life I promised myself when we first moved here. I have 12 hornets' stings to thank for that. No wonder you hate me. But I am determined. I cannot stand your attacks any more and after one blazing row I slam my head against a wall. I don't know what else to do. You are threatening to run away. Again.

"Don't bother," I yell, my head pounding. "I'll go." I walk out, slamming the front door behind me. The problem now is that your dad and I like our life here – so do your sisters – and we want to live it fully. You hate everything about it and see it through a veil of vengeful fury. I need to protect our life just as much as your recovery needs protecting. There has been enough collateral damage. I don't think you are able to see that yet. I am equally terrified about what will happen when you do.

As I walk, I remember. It isn't the first time I've hit my head against a wall. You were six, maybe seven. Two hours after first putting you to bed, I eventually closed your door. You sat bolt up, immediately alert, the door needed to be at a specific place and I had blown it. I was tired and crotchety, I wanted a glass of wine, I wanted to watch telly and I'd run out of patience. I snapped. I said something mean. I can't remember what I said, but it scared you and now you're wide awake.

"You did that!" you shouted. You were right. I had said something scary because I was cross with you for being scared. That's fucked up. That's why I slammed my head against the wall, I was frustrated with you and furious with myself. The following week, I booked myself into a fast-track, pull-no-punches therapy workshop weekend. It was brutal. But it helped. About 250 people with various, often hideous, life experiences, whittled down to a universal fear and a universal desire. As individuals, we weren't good enough and whatever we had, we wanted more. The human condition, seen collectively. It was almost funny – how we cling to our stories, how we let them drag us down, how we need to get out of the way of ourselves.

The shingle beach crunches beneath my feet. I need that clarity and perspective again. My sisters had been urging me to find someone to talk to, but I had felt too exhausted to talk about it while we were living in it and my view of therapy was pretty low, but I clearly need help to get out of this miserable Roxy and Gay story. I dial a number of a therapist that I've had for some time but resisted calling. By some miracle, she has an appointment immediately. By another, she's one mile from where I am presently standing. I say a prayer to our guardian angel, still looking out for you.

I sink into the yellow sofa and tell her I'm fine. Obviously, she sees right through me and we go to work. It all comes gushing out. Hours of it.

"What's exhausting is trying to work out, with split-second timing, whether the 'downs' we hit are a cry for help or a resurgence of the psychosis. Is it poor health or poor behaviour? It's like standing in quicksand. The wrong move, and I go under. Do nothing, and I sink anyway."

"It is never either/or," she says. "It is always 'and' and 'both'."

Huh?

She explains that woven into the exceptional psychological pain you experience, there will be bog-standard teenage crap. Equally, woven into standard teenage pain will be real psychological challenges.

"The ups and downs are exhausting," I lament.

She draws a wavy line on a piece of paper. "There are going to be ups and downs," she says. "But eventually the downs – though they feel cataclysmic at the time – cease to be as low as they were, and the ups, though they feel small, get steadily higher." The wiggly line is climbing up the page. "The argument this morning feels like you're back to the beginning, but you aren't." Her pen rests halfway up her line of peaks and troughs. I can see it! We are climbing out of the pit of despair. I feel a tremor of something, something a bit like … hope.

"There will be more mountains to climb," she says. "This will be true for the rest of your daughter's life. It will be true of yours too. But you get swifter and stronger and better able to climb them."

This exceptionally skilled woman renews my faith in therapy and gives me the courage to trust you to the same process with a therapist of your own. We had both been burned, but we are both rewarded for trying again.

And and both becomes the mantra that carries me through the rest of your school year. *And and both* allows me to respond to the pain without reacting to the behaviour (most of the time). *And and both* gets me out of the quicksand and back on to terra firma. My therapist gives me the confidence to parent again. She gives me the confidence to reclaim my place in the house and the world. I wasn't the best mother, but I was good enough. The strength that had got us through was becoming a weakness. I have to let go. She gives me the courage to do that and to trust you can find your own footholds and safety ropes and that you will not hate me and you will not die.

It is one massive fucking leap of faith.

HEADACHE

I am on the sofa back at home. I have been here for almost three weeks now. My GCSEs are in a month and I cannot get off this sofa. I go for a walk every day and sometimes I talk to a new therapist you found for me. Mostly, though, I just lie on this sofa watching TV and drawing cubes. I crashed a while ago. I guess that I sort of knew that the life I was living wasn't sustainable; the 12 hours of studying – I thought that I could make it through to after exams, but my mind and my body have given up on me. I am weak. Walking up the stairs is exhausting. We are back to you and I spending days in the kitchen, except you have a life now, and that hurts even more. What a selfish prick I am, hating you for being happy. We aren't even arguing. I am too tired to argue; we just don't speak. The dog is curled up next to me and I am wearing the pyjamas that I put on four days ago and haven't taken off. My hair is a tangled mess on top of my head, just one big dreadlock. The thought of battling with it is so exhausting, so I am just letting it get worse and worse.

I have an ice pack on my forehead because I have been getting these excruciating headaches. My eyebrows ache all the time, I rub them to try ease the pain, and sometimes I can't stop myself pulling the hairs out. My head feels like this heavy weight that my body cannot support any more. Keeping my eyes open hurts and I lie down most of the time.

Dad is angry at me for missing so much school. I don't think that is particularly fair – I can't be accused of not taking school seriously, I got my mock results back recently and I got A*s in every subject. Surely you both realize that if I could get off this sofa, then I would. Getting through these exams is the most important thing in the world to me right now. You think I don't know that I need GCSEs to prove everyone wrong and get my life back on track? I CANNOT GET OFF THIS SOFA. Everything is too heavy.

There is so much that I need to process and think about, but I keep distracting myself so that I don't have to engage. How am I ever supposed to come to terms with the photos? Those images and those positions still haunt me. Why did I send them? That question really makes my head spin. Part of it was the thrill, the excitement. It was exciting at the start. I was so flattered. Roxy, the nerdy, weird girl who had never been considered "hot", was getting all this attention. Maybe it was nothing more profound than that. Perhaps there is no reason to dig deeper, there is no fundamental issue that I was dealing with. It is possible that I was just a stupid teenage girl who wanted some attention, was flattered when she got it, and thought that sending photos was the only way to keep it. I look back on other pictures of me from that time and my heart breaks for that girl. I look so young. What am I saying? I *was* so young. Even with the straightened hair and dark eyelashes and push-up bras, I look my age: 13 years old. When I look at the photos, it feels so wrong that those guys even wanted them. I was a child with a chubby round baby face. I've looked back at the photos that Alex and I took together. They almost look quite innocent, like a toddler dressing up in her mum's high heels and jewellery for the first time. They aren't innocent, though; we thought we looked hot, and the guys thought we looked hot. I can't really understand it. It wasn't two silly girls dressing up and messing around in their rooms – it was somehow darker than that because it wasn't for us, it was for them. Or maybe I just remember it like that now because of everything that happened after. I don't know.

I want to explain why I did it so that young girls don't do it any more. I mean, I don't think there is a problem with sending photographs if you are an adult in a relationship with another adult and you make that decision knowing the potential risks. If you are in a long-distance relationship, then I understand why you might.

But to the 13-, 14-, 15- year-old girls: if you are sending these photographs, then you probably think that there is no way what happened to me will happen to you. I thought that too. I had heard stories of people whose lives were ruined, but that wasn't enough to stop me. I promise you it is not worth it. It may make you feel sexy and grown-up, empowered and wanted – and I know I wouldn't have listened to anyone who spouted this shit at me when I was 13, so I doubt you will take this on board – but it isn't worth it. The fact is that these boys could find images of much more attractive women online very easily, so I worry that it is more about having control over a girl. You are a girl, so don't kid yourself into thinking you are a woman. The moment they have those photos, they own you. I think that is what appeals to them much more than the images themselves. Power. The thing is, I did it. I sent the photos and then they were used against me. I still feel disgusting.

*

I am in the middle of a boring episode of a TV show I have watched too many times. Dad storms into the room and shouts.

"Roxy, you cannot spend the rest of your life on this sofa. You have to go to school just like everybody else your age in this country."

I don't even respond. He has completely missed the point. He storms back to the kitchen and I hear him shout to you,

"I cannot do this, Gay, I do not know what to do."

You come into the room next.

"Enough! You signed up to this, this is what you wanted, so get off the sofa and go back to school."

"I can't."

"You have to."

"My head hurts."

"I will take you to a doctor about the headaches, but you cannot spend another week at home. You need to be at school."

"I don't want to go."

"Tough shit. You're going back."

Two days later, I go back to school and I start studying again. You gave me a figurative bitch-slap and it got me off the sofa. You are the only person who could've done that. I take a lot of pain killers for the constant pain in my face and head, but at least I am revising again and going to lessons. I have some really amazing teachers here. They think I am smart and capable and they are trying to make me see that. I am struggling to accept that when these people look at me, they don't see a slut who went crazy. I am suspicious. My English, Biology and French teachers are particularly amazing. They really help me see what my brain can truly do.

*

I am sitting in a shisha bar with friends. Like, actual people from school. This incredible girl kept inviting me to sit with her at lunch and knocking on my door to say she was going out with some friends and asking if I would like to come. I dismissed all her generous attempts to get me out of my room. I said that I had too much work to do. My extreme anxiety about socializing definitely came across as rudeness. I would beat myself up horrendously every time I said no to her invitations. Anyway, one day she walked in and said:

"That is it. You are coming out with me right now. There is more to life than studying."

And now I am here, and I am laughing. They tease me for being so studious, and it is the nicest thing I have ever been teased about.

SPAGHETTI

You do find your own footholds and you learn to tie your own safety ropes. They come in the form of a few special people: new friends from college, old friends from school who re-emerge, and a couple who never deserted you in the first place. Precious friends. Lifers, I hope. Enough to have a party. My first teen party. I stand hidden in the dark and watch out of a side window as you and your friends pass the obligatory red plastic tumblers around, spill outside laughing loudly, surreptitiously smoke, wobble and dance. In the countryside, the kids tend to stay over; roll mats and sleeping bags are essential party kit. I am determined to separate the girls from the boys. They have a curfew, so at 1 a.m., I go in and pull out the girls.

Upstairs, there is a bit of commotion. One of your oldest friends is kneeling over the loo. She looks up at me. Her long blonde hair is being held back by another girl.

"Sorry, Gay," she says, pitifully. We put her to bed on her side. Note to self: don't serve spaghetti bolognese to teens.

One of your canniest girlfriends gets round my curfew, climbs out of a downstairs window and goes back to the boys. You know who you are! I don't mind. Actually, I rather admire the chutzpah.

In the morning, bedraggled kids emerge for tea and toast. They will never know how happy it made us, hosting a gaggle of boys and girls who were taking the piss out of each other, laughing, leaving crumbs everywhere, lounging about. You have been up for two hours working and now that the beached teens have roused themselves you have donned the Marigolds and set off with the bucket and mop to clean up. You are not an ordinary teen and I love you for it.

When you hit bumps, you have a phenomenal therapist to work through things with. You also start to exercise, maybe a bit obsessively, but exercise runs the excess adrenaline out of your system, so it works. You discover walking and audiobooks. You take up songwriting and play the guitar. I could listen to you and your sisters sing forever. Music helps, nature helps. Your GCSE results are staggeringly good and you choose maths, chemistry and biology for your A levels. You'll always have something to feed your inquisitive brain. Your work ethic is exceptional. When all else fails, as sometimes it does, there is always a soppy polar bear-white Labrador to curl up with and wait out the storm.

It doesn't matter what the footholds are, what matters is that we find them – one foothold at a time. They are precious. They save lives. Mine are a few special people, one phenomenal therapist, yoga, chakra work, sea swimming, sunsets, my sisters, my husband and long walks with a soppy polar bear-white Labrador.

I think about the people who helped us get to where we are today, whether that was merely a moment or those who were in it for the long-haul, a chicken pie, a rescue mission, a shoulder, or a random person sharing their hard-won wisdom. One retired mental health nurse told me it is remarkable what young people can experience and still go on to thrive and what happened to us was not so abnormal. She told me of children in the foetal position on the floor unable to function – check – then seeing them five years later, remarkable young people, packing up supplies for adventures abroad – check, as it turned out.

I believe there is a common denominator to every person who helps us: they have experienced life at the sharp end and survived. They all give us something to take on our journey. They had been through the portal and were there to catch us when life chewed us up and spat us out. We landed in a heap on the floor and they pulled us up, one by one, and without judgement, were strong enough to hold on to us until we were able to hold on ourselves. That is what resilience means to me: it is being strong enough to help others until they are strong enough to help themselves so that they are strong enough to help others until they are strong enough to help themselves ... and so it continues. You are helped up so you can help others up after you.

Generosity of spirit is the greatest strength of all.
Happiness is the greatest revenge.
Courage is essential.

BEER PONG

"What if nobody turns up?"

I am having a party. I now have a handful of amazing friends –
some new, some who have stuck with me all the way through this
shitshow. They have persuaded me that I should try to have fun
again. It terrifies me. Maybe I don't think that I deserve fun, maybe
I am scared that if I start having fun again then I am proving
everybody right, maybe I don't trust myself to have fun and not go
back to that person I used to be. I don't know but I am doing this
anyway – and I am also genuinely worried that nobody is going
to turn up. I don't really have enough friends to have a party but
I've told everyone to bring people. I want to meet new people
and reconnect with the ones who fell out of my life.

I have been going back and forth about whether or not to
do this for days. Nobody is going to turn up. You are bored of
this conversation, which I guess is fair enough. I don't say this
to you because I am an idiot but I am so grateful that you are
being so relaxed about this. I know that you are making it all as
easy as possible for me; you want me to have friends and have
fun and be happy. You know that I have missed out on a lot of
my teenage years and you are helping me start to make up for
it. I am grateful and I don't tell you.

This party is driving me crazy, so I am grasping for any form
of distraction. That is basically how my life works now: a balance

between distracting myself and teaching myself how to sit with my feelings and manage them. Distraction is obviously not a sustainable solution, and I know that, but I can't be fighting with my brain all the time – it is exhausting and I will break. So sometimes I just have to watch TV and make a collage. I can't do only one or the other because that does not distract me enough. I have to do at least two things at the same time. Then, when I am feeling stronger, I try to do just one thing and sit with myself. I scrub the floor with a toothbrush, getting all the dirt out of the little cracks. I suppose it is sort of my version of mindfulness. They say that the things that help with anxiety are yoga, breathing and exercise, but I really think that you have to find your own thing. Lots of things don't work – I hate yoga. I know that I cannot be left alone with my thoughts for long periods of time, so I distract myself when I need to and challenge myself to work with my brain when I feel up to it.

I know that I sound very put together and like I have this sorted. In reality, what this means is that I've worked out that when I start to spiral into a hyperventilating, crying, screaming, restless mess, the best way to calm down is to distract myself by doing lots of things at the same time. After a while, I realized that the distractions are only a short-term solution, but crucial nonetheless. Once I have calmed down to a reasonably sane place, then I can start to negotiate with my stubborn brain.

The party is today and I feel sick. I have a plan to make a joke about the photos or about dropping out of school early on in the evening. I want them to feel like they don't have to walk on eggshells around me. They need to know that I am not a fragile, emotional mess who could break at any moment. I get dressed up and put on make-up and a crop top.

This does not make you a slut, Roxy.

People do turn up. Thank fuck. I have a drink and I dance and I chat and I feel amazing. These people don't care about what happened last year. I can be fun and funny and ask interesting questions. I can do this.

By the time everyone wakes up, I have done two hours of revision. I am hungover and I don't want to work, but I know that if I don't, then the self-loathing later will be consuming. When everyone wakes up, they sprawl across the sofas talking about what happened the night before. I cannot do the lounging about and chatting, my brain just tells me that I am wasting time when I should be doing something productive. So I vacuum and scrub the surfaces around them, wearing my rubber gloves. They take the piss, obviously, and that is okay. It is good. They like me despite all the messiness and I don't have to hide.

MORE BEAUTIFUL FOR HAVING BEEN BROKEN (BUT I WISH YOU'D NEVER BEEN BROKEN)

On your eighteenth birthday, your dad and I hug each other and burst into tears. They are tears of pride. We are so proud of your climb out of the well. We feel joy, because you are surrounded by friends; relief, because you are alive; and exhaustion, because it took a great deal of hard work to get you here. There is a touch of shock and awe that we made it. We're not naive – we know not to get complacent – but we take that moment and celebrate it.

You took hit, after hit, after hit. The photos damaged you, but the blame broke you and psychosis took over. First it drew an inaccessible veil of darkness between you and the rest of the world and in that disassociated state we, the people who love you, couldn't reach you. What did follow you into the darkness was other people's cruelty, echoing and amplifying all the self-loathing until you were brought to your knees.

I hope you know now that you were a child who deserved to be protected by us, by the school and by the professionals who should have made it clear from the very first moment that this was not your fault. You have punished yourself long enough. I know you take responsibility for your actions, but it is time to protect that little girl from any more blame. We have always loved you and will always love you, I am so sorry that I didn't stop this from happening to you. I will carry that regret to my grave.

To reflect what you have been through, I choose a piece of Japanese pottery mended through a process called kintsugi for your birthday. Cracked pots are put back together with gold lacquer. They are broken and then they are recreated, reformed, rebuilt. I wish with all my heart that you hadn't had to break, I wish I knew then what I know now. You have gleaned so much, you have grown so much, you are an exceptional 18-year-old, and more beautiful for having been broken.

When you were very little, we were one unit, then we broke and then we decided to write a book together. We were at loggerheads within minutes. We could barely be in the same room, so different were each other's experiences of what had happened. Then lockdown happened and, with your A levels cancelled, you had to come home. You disappeared into one room to write, I into another. Only when we were done did we read the other's version and start to understand. Writing this book has given us the chance to mend despite feeling smashed and beyond repair when we started. Two pots, one story.

It is a privilege to be your mother. You have taught me more than you will ever know. I guess the hardest lessons are the ones we don't want to learn, but we do need to learn them. Everyday sexism, #MeToo, Reclaim These Streets, Everyone's Invited – so many voices desperate to communicate that we are collectively getting something fatally wrong. Dr B told me when you were ill that mental health issues get worse incrementally if left untreated. Children aren't born schizophrenics. Perpetrators aren't born either. They are made. The boys who did this to you could have made different choices and none of this would have happened. Why did they do it? I've searched and searched for a plausible answer. When I found it, it was staggeringly simple. Why do they do it? Because they can.

I watch you look after your remarkable brain every day. I watch you choose to make the decision to do that even when it feels impossibly hard. Intrusive, critical thoughts are exhausting and an empty mind is impossible. All any of us can do is attempt to control the thoughts and the feelings our minds evoke rather than be controlled by them. Turn our thinking from destructive to productive. It isn't easy – none of this is easy – but I think it is worth it. I think of your brain as a prancing, powerful stallion, skittish but strong; you have had to learn how to ride it. It has repeatedly bucked you off and bolted in dangerous directions, but when you hit your stride, it will give you the ride of your life.

That ride starts now.

PURA VIDA

As I'm sat here writing this, I still cannot believe that we have gotten to this point. Mama, we've written a fucking book. We go out for drinks together, and we laugh, and we tease each other for the things that used to cause month-long arguments. That is the thing that makes me most proud. The realization that I had to stop expecting you to be the perfect mother that I thought I needed, that I thought I deserved – a blank slate of a person whose only purpose was to support. I know that this sounds obvious, but I sort of didn't realize that you had your own complex personality, your own messy internal world, your own battles with an intricate brain.

You will always say silly, hurtful things that you haven't thought through, especially when you feel even remotely attacked. Now I can laugh at your careless insensitivity instead of taking your comments and holding on to them, letting them eat me up and using them to build the case that I have an awful mother. I used it as an excuse to not deal with the fact that my unhappiness was caused by myself, and my brain. I have an incredible mother, I am so, so lucky. I love that you go away and properly think about conversations you've had with people, you ponder and deliberate until you have formed the perfect response. Your advice is never lazy – it is wise and you are so generous with your time. You will listen when someone needs to be listened to, advise them when they need help, and bitch-slap them when they need a serious kick up the arse. I have more respect for you than you could possibly know.

On top of this, you have taught me how to see the best in people and how to be strong and generous. You stuck by me for so many years when all I did was use you as a punchbag. No matter how awful I was, you kept believing that there was a good person somewhere inside. You have somehow taught me to use my destructive, controlling brain as a force for good. Also, and I think this is the most important, you have taught me how to have as much fun as possible. You have this incredible ability to walk into a room and make it light up, this infectious energy. As Dad said, "Everybody bloody loves Gay." That is so true. I used to think that this was because they didn't know the real you, but actually it was me who didn't know the real you because I was so set on you being the awful person I had created in my head. I now know how lucky I am to have been blessed with a mum who dropped everything to take care of me when I couldn't take care of myself.

I feel sorry for anybody who has to listen to you and I talk. We can practically read each other's minds, so our conversations are just a whole load of unfinished sentences and vague pronouns.

"Let's tell thingamabob to get that thing from that place and then we've got to finish that stuff."

"Yep."

"Then let's do—"

"Uh-huh, and don't forget the—"

"Yeah, of course."

We both know exactly what the other means and everybody around us is just desperately confused. I know that connection isn't always a good thing, but it is immensely powerful – something to be cautious of but also so grateful for.

I know that I am still cold and sarcastic, and not always the kindest, but I love you with all my heart. I am so sorry for everything. I do not know what I would do without you.

For your fiftieth birthday, I made you a film of your greatest friends reading "Desiderata", just as you used to recite it to me, we leave you, the reader, with the last few lines.

... in the noisy confusion of life, keep peace in your soul.
With all its sham, drudgery and broken dreams, it is still a
beautiful world. Be cheerful. Strive to be happy.

Postscript

WHEN YOU LOSE IT: AN ESSAY FOR MENTAL HEALTH AWARENESS WEEK, 8–12 MAY 2017

200,000 years ago, fear was vital to the survival of the species we call *Homo sapiens*, it got us to where we are today. A rustle in the grass, YOU ARE NOT SAFE – RUN – a predator is coming to get you. No matter if it turned out to be the wind, better to run from the wind than stay and be devoured. It was also essential that we remembered all the times we stumbled into dangerous territory, heard that rustle and got away. Remembering the bad stuff increased our chances of survival. Humans are really good at remembering the bad stuff.

Every single fear, real or imagined, gets the required injection of hormones from the adrenal cortex in the brain that first tells you to RUN – YOU ARE NOT SAFE, then allows you to KEEP ON RUNNING. Humans can't escape predators on speed; instead, we are given the ability to react immediately to danger and then endure a long escape. You'll know the feeling: your heart starts to pump fast, delivering oxygen to the blood and that blood to the muscles, your sweat glands get ready to cool you down, your breath quickens to suck in more air, your stomach constricts – digestion is no use now, you need all your energy elsewhere – you are now primed to run about 5 miles if you really needed to. The only problem is, we are firmly on top of the food chain now; we have dominated our world and changed it. There are no predators in the long grass. Or are there?

Exam results, performance pressures, popularity pressures, to like or not to like, sibling rivalry, body image, death, divorce, ill health, bad news, important matches, world events, injustice,

envy, financial worries, job security, extremism, pandemics …
the list of things to fear goes on and on and we invent new ones
every day, left swipe, right swipe. It is easy to imagine feeling
worried all the time, yet we still only have one way to respond.
RUN. RUN FAST. RUN FAR AND KEEP ON RUNNING
BECAUSE YOU ARE NOT SAFE!

Now remember that bit about remembering the bad bits,
the bits to be afraid of, and you have a biochemical superstorm
building in the brain. What you need to be able to do in that
state is switch off and fall into a deep restorative sleep, during
which the brain regulates the multitude of hormones that affect
mood and the medial prefrontal cortex can sift through the
things that are real worries and discard the ones that aren't. But
you can't. You have 200 miles of adrenaline racing around your
system when in fact you haven't left your desk.

So now add the fear of not sleeping. Absolutely guaranteed to
keep you awake. The next day is a challenge, concentration easily
wanes. The tired brain picks up signals and magnifies it. The brain
becomes hyperalert to threat and senses danger everywhere.

Eventually the circuit breaks.

The brain rewires to the locus coeruleus. The locus coeruleus
secretes norepinephrine, the precursor to full fight, flight or
freeze mode. The brain is now actively keeping itself awake as a
means of survival. Hallucinations are the external manifestations
of all those feelings of fear that the brain, without the protective work of sleep, simply cannot deal with. It has effectively
tripped. Without the LSD.

And if you can't run away, if you are trapped, the brain will
provide other more sinister ways to escape. It will whisper over
and over that your friends and family will be better off without
you. I don't know why it does this, but it is not true. It has been

calculated that on average, every suicide negatively impacts 134 people for the rest of their lives. Ignore the voice, get help.

It can happen to anyone. The CIA used sleep deprivation as torture in Guantanamo Bay Prison after 9/11. It left no marks and got results fast. The intelligence, however, was unreliable, and after several sleepless nights the prisoners were experiencing terrifying visual and auditory misperceptions. Their testimony could not be counted on and they'd become a danger to themselves. Look up Operation Sandman if you don't believe me.

So as it turns out, sleep is the key. Thank goodness teenagers are so well known for having healthy sleep patterns ...

We can trick the reptilian brain into believing it has outrun the beast by actively elevating the heart rate for 20 minutes. Now hit the ground and give me 20! Burpees, anyone?

Alternatively, breathing and grounding exercises can anchor you back in the present. Don't recommend you use a raisin, though.

Perhaps all I can offer you is this instead. You are not alone. Everyone has an internal voice. It's the one that just said, "*I* don't."

Find your way to switch your brain from overproducing heart-racing adrenaline so it can start secreting the nice stuff like dopamine and serotonin, better still melatonin ... because trust me when I tell you, sleep is the key.

THE LAST WORD

God, I hate it when you bang on about sleep.

The End